THE POCKET GUIDE TO VITAMINS

ANGELA DOWDEN

PAN BOOKS

First published 2013 by Pan Books
an imprint of Pan Macmillan, a division of Macmillan Publishers Limited
Pan Macmillan, 20 New Wharf Road, London N1 9RR
Basingstoke and Oxford
Associated companies throughout the world
www.panmacmillan.com

ISBN 978-1-4472-5847-6

1 3 5 7 9 8 6 4 2

A CIP catalogue record for this book is available from the British Library.

Designed and typeset by seagulls.net
Printed by CPI Group (UK) Ltd, Croydon, CR0 4YY

Visit **www.panmacmillan.com** to read more about all our books
and to buy them. You will also find features, author interviews and
news of any author events, and you can sign up for e-newsletters
so that you're always first to hear about our new releases.

CONTENTS

INTRODUCTION

We all know that a good diet is vital to staying fit and healthy, and that eating well is the best way to get all the vitamins and minerals that we need. But with busy schedules, processed foods and entrenched (and sometimes undesirable) diet and lifestyle habits, can you be sure you are getting enough essential nutrients for your needs?

These days, major vitamin and mineral deficiencies (at least in the fortunate West) are very rare, but more minor nutrient deficiencies can still have the potential to undermine our health. For example, sub-optimal levels of vitamin D might not cause anything as dramatic as bendy bones, but could lead to more vague symptoms such as fatigue, depression and joint pain. And marginally deficient levels of vitamin A won't lead to blindness (as more severe deficiencies do in developing countries), but may lead to a weakened immune system and problematic skin.

But how can you know which vitamins and minerals you are most likely to be short of, and which diet will best cover your nutrient needs? Would snacking more intelligently, eating more oily fish, or avoiding too many processed foods make things better, or could you still benefit from a supplement? And, more to the point, if you do decide to pop a pill – around one in three of us already do – which one is right for you, with all those vitamins and supplements shouting to us from the chemist, supermarket and internet 'shelves'?

These, and other topics, are the issues we cover in this pocket guide to vitamins, minerals and other potentially health-giving supplements such as fish oils, herbs and probiotics. Our aim is to cover the basics of this complex and ever-evolving branch of nutrition science in an accessible, dip-in-and-out sort of way. This is neither a pill-pushing guide, nor a book that complacently assumes we're all replete with vitamins just because scurvy is no longer rife. Instead we aim to present the available evidence to help you decide whether you are getting all the nutrients you need, whether a supplement might help, and how to choose the right product if you do go down that route.

We hope you'll be able to use this handy reference to help improve your well-being, and to find the right diet and health solutions for you.

Good health and good reading!

VITAMINS AND MINERALS: THE BASICS

WHAT ARE VITAMINS AND MINERALS ANYWAY?

Unlike protein, carbohydrates and fat, vitamins and minerals do not provide us with energy (calories), and are not needed in large amounts. In fact, some vitamins and minerals are only required in daily quantities that could fit on a pinhead, yet their impact on health is profound. Most act as facilitators in key biological processes, such as those that drive energy production, muscle contraction and the transmission of nerve impulses. If you think of your body as a stately home, the vitamins are like tiny domestic servants, scurrying around to stoke the fires, turn on the lights and maintain the internal fixtures and fittings, whereas minerals tend to be the more structural stuff in the building, like bricks and mortar, without which the whole edifice would fall apart.

Vitamins can also be distinguished from minerals on the basis of their chemistry. Vitamins are 'organic' – containing carbon and hydrogen – and are largely manufactured by plants and bacteria. Minerals, on the other hand, are 'inorganic' (not containing carbon or hydrogen), and originate in the earth's crust. With the exception of vitamin D, our bodies do not have the ability to make vitamins or minerals, which is why obtaining them through diet is so important.

VITAMINS

Thirteen substances have been classified as vitamins. These are vitamin A, vitamin D, vitamin E, vitamin K, vitamin C and eight B vitamins. Vitamins A, D, E and K are fat soluble, which means that reserves of them can be stored in the body and a consistent daily supply is not essential. The B and C vitamins, however, are water soluble, and need to be replenished very regularly as they do not stay in the body very long. Any excess is excreted via the urine, and the body can only handle small intakes at any one time.

MINERALS

Minerals are split into 'macro' minerals (such as calcium, magnesium and potassium), which are needed in larger amounts by the body, and 'trace' minerals, which, as the name suggests, are only needed in tiny quantities. Despite only being needed in such small amounts, trace minerals include such vital nutrients as iron and zinc.

TINY BUT IMPORTANT

Most vitamins, minerals and other active ingredients that might be found in a supplement are measured in milligrams (mg) or micrograms (µg, or mcg). A milligram is one thousandth of a gram, which sounds teeny enough. But a microgram is one thousandth of that amount again (or just one *millionth* of a gram). To give you two practical examples of how milligrams and micrograms translate, the RDA, Recommended Daily Allowance, of calcium – 800mg – equals one fifth of the weight of a level teaspoon of sugar. The RDA of vitamin B12 – just 2.5 micrograms – weighs only one thousandth of the weight of one grain of sand!

DAILY REQUIREMENTS

In 1991, the UK government's Committee on the Medical Aspect of Food Policy (since disbanded) published comprehensive daily vitamin and mineral consumption guidelines for both sexes and across all age groups. Known as RNIs (Reference Nutrient Intakes) they were defined as 'the amount of the nutrient that is enough, or more than enough for about 97% of people in a group'. RNIs continue to be used in UK health and nutrition policy and are still considered a largely valid estimate of how much each population group needs to meet its daily needs. Throughout this book, we'll generally refer to EU RDAs (Recommended Daily Allowances) rather than UK RNIs, however, as RDAs are the figures that are currently required to be used on food and food supplement packaging across Europe. EU RDAs are identical in definition to UK RNIs, except that they were devised for use across countries and comprise one average figure for an average adult, rather than being broken down into figures for several age groups and both sexes.

RDAs are the most up-to-date available guide of how much of a particular nutrient you should aim to consume daily to meet your basic needs. But it is worth bearing in mind that variations in genetics, body size and general state of health mean

GOING FORWARD

As of late 2013, the European Food Safety Authority will again be reviewing vitamin and mineral requirements, and is due to publish updated figures that will replace Recommended Daily Allowances. These will be called Dietary Reference Values, so in the future you'll see 'DRV' rater than 'RDA' on supplement labels.

that the level of a vitamin or mineral that is *optimal* can differ a lot from person to person. And given that recommendations vary around the world, it's best to use them as a guideline only.

THE RDAS AND RNIS OF VITAMINS AND MINERALS

VITAMIN OR MINERAL	EU RDA	UK RNI (MEN)	UK RNI (WOMEN)
Vitamin A	800µg	700µg	600µg (700µg in pregnancy, 950µg whilst breast-feeding)
Thiamin (Vitamin B1)	1.1mg	1mg (0.9mg over age 50)	0.8mg (1mg whilst breast-feeding)
Riboflavin (Vitamin B2)	1.4mg	1.3mg	1.1mg (1.4mg in pregnancy, 1.6mg whilst breast-feeding)
Niacin (Vitamin B3)	16mg	17mg (16mg over age 50)	13mg (15mg whilst breast-feeding, 12mg over age 50)
Pantothenic Acid (Vitamin B5)	6mg	—	—
Vitamin B6	1.4mg	1.4mg	1.2mg
Biotin (also known as Vitamin B7)	50µg	—	—
Folic Acid (also known as Vitamin B9)	200µg	200µg	200µg (600µg in first three months of pregnancy, 260µg whilst breast-feeding)
Vitamin B12	2.5µg	1.5µg	1.5µg (2µg whilst breast-feeding)
Vitamin C	80mg	40mg	40mg (50mg during pregnancy, 70mg whilst breast-feeding)

VITAMIN OR MINERAL	EU RDA	UK RNI (MEN)	UK RNI (WOMEN)
Vitamin D	5µg	10µg for over 65s*	10µg in pregnancy, whilst breast-feeding and for over 65s*
Vitamin E	12mg	—	—
Vitamin K	75µg	—	—
Potassium	2000mg	3500mg	3500mg
Calcium	800mg	700mg	700mg (1250mg whilst breast-feeding)
Phosphorus	700mg	550mg	550mg (990mg whilst breast-feeding)
Magnesium	375mg	300mg	270mg (320mg whilst breast-feeding)
Iron	14mg	8.7mg	14.8mg (8.7mg over age 50)
Zinc	10mg	9.5mg	7mg (13mg whilst breast-feeding)
Copper	1mg	1.2mg	1.2mg (1.5mg whilst breast-feeding)
Manganese	2mg	—	—
Selenium	55µg	75µg	60µg (75µg whilst breast-feeding)
Molybdenum	50µg	—	—
Chromium	40µg	—	—
Iodine	150µg	140µg	140µg

— RNI not established.

* Assumed that dietary vitamin D not required in younger adults as can be formed from sunlight.

A DIET TO MEET YOUR VITAMIN NEEDS

Without doubt, the best way for us to obtain our nutrients is through eating real food. No matter how well formulated, a vitamin or mineral supplement can never mimic the rich diversity of nutrients, antioxidants and phyto (plant) chemicals provided by a healthy, balanced diet. But what sort of diet should we be eating? Nutrition scientists may disagree on the minor points of what constitutes healthy eating, but not on the fundamentals. For example, there is general agreement that a varied diet is critical to achieving nutritional adequacy, and that including foods from across all food groups (proteins, carbohydrates, dairy products and healthy fats) will make it easier to meet vitamin and mineral needs. Below is a whistle-stop tour of the food groups and a guide to how much of each we should be eating to cover essential nutrient needs:

FRUIT AND VEGETABLES

Provide: vitamin C, folic acid, vitamins A, E and K, plus other antioxidants and phytochemicals
As an ideal, around half of each meal should be made up of fruit and veg, with somewhat more vegetables being consumed than fruit. The bigger point, though, is to eat as many varieties as you can manage, and to choose across the colour spectrum (including oranges, greens, reds and purples), as differently coloured fruit and veg tend to have different nutrient profiles. To make it easier, frozen, tinned, juiced and dried types of fruit and veg all count.

QUALITY CARBOHYDRATES

Provide: B vitamins, iron and magnesium
Many people have cut down on bread, pasta, rice and other carbohydrates (carbs for short) in recent years, having heard

reports that they are fattening or otherwise bad for health. Meanwhile, government healthy eating guidelines (which many regard as out of date) still urge us to eat plenty of these starchy foods. A look at the latest evidence suggests we should probably be doing something in the middle: filling a modest quarter of our plates with carb-rich foods, but making sure they are as nutrient dense as possible. The ones that will particularly help maximise your vitamin and mineral intake include pulses (such as baked beans, chickpeas, lentils, kidney beans and hummus), seeded and grainy wholemeal breads, and fortified breakfast cereals.

DAIRY PRODUCTS

Provide: calcium, iodine and riboflavin
Not everyone agrees that dairy is an essential food group, but it's an inarguable fact that dairy products are a key provider of calcium and iodine for most Britons. Certainly, eating two portions of dairy (milk, yoghurt or cheese) daily will make it much more likely that you'll meet your needs for these two nutrients when on a typical Western diet. For people with dairy intolerances or allergies, dairy alternatives like soya, rice or almond milk are fortified with as much calcium as dairy milk, but won't be as rich a source of iodine.

LEAN PROTEINS

Provide: iron, zinc, thiamin, niacin and iodine
Protein sources such as chicken, lean red meat, offal, white fish and seafood (or vegetarian alternatives such as soya beans, eggs, tofu and quorn) should ideally be served in the same quantities as healthy carbs, filling around a quarter of your plate. Choosing a variety of these different protein sources will maximise the range of vitamins and minerals you obtain.

OILY FISH, NUTS AND OTHER
SOURCES OF HEALTHY FATS

Provide: vitamin D, omega-3 fats, iron, zinc, selenium, calcium and vitamin E

Eating at least one weekly portion of oily fish (canned or fresh salmon, sardines, mackerel or herring), and adding a small handful, sprinkle or drizzle of nuts, seeds, avocado or vegetable oil to your daily diet, will provide important omega-3 oils, plus fat-soluble vitamins D and E. As well as providing vitamin E, many nuts and seeds are also great sources of minerals, including zinc and calcium.

CONSERVING VITAMINS AND MINERALS

Many vitamins are vulnerable to attack through heat, air, moisture and light. By contrast, minerals are quite stable, but can be leached away in cooking water. Try these tips to preserve more nutrients:

- Buy fruit and vegetables little and often, keep cool, and eat within a few days. Frozen fruit and veg retain their vitamins well and are good choices, especially if you can only shop irregularly. There's no need to be sniffy about canned food either, as canning processes have become more sophisticated over the years so a higher percentage of nutrients is retained.
- If you buy bottled milk, don't leave it on the doorstep, as sunlight destroys riboflavin (vitamin B2).
- Cook vegetables for the minimum amount of time (so they are still crunchy). Steaming, quick stir-frying and micro-waving are good cooking methods to retain vitamins. If

you boil veg, use the minimum amount of water, introduce the vegetables straight to the hot water and use a tight-fitting lid. Pressure cooking uses higher temperatures but can still retain vitamins well, as long as you don't overcook.

- Avoid leaving cut vegetables exposed to air, heat or light, don't soak them prior to cooking, and never use bicarbonate of soda to keep vegetables green (it completely destroys vitamin C).

- Use cooking water and meat juices for soups and gravies, as you'll retain some of the iron, zinc and magnesium leached into them.

- Larger chunks of fruits and vegetables, rather than fine pieces, will also lose fewer vitamins as there is less surface area exposed to air. Try to avoid peeling wherever possible, as in many cases vitamins are most highly concentrated just under the skin.

- Use the absorption method for cooking brown grains. When brown rice is cooked in the minimum amount of water, figures show that a lot less thiamin (vitamin B1) is leached out than when cooked in a large amount of liquid.

- Once food is cooked try to eat it straight away, because keeping food hot can destroy vitamins. Food standing for 15 minutes may result in a 25% loss of vitamin C, whilst food kept hot for 90 minutes, such as in a canteen, loses 75%.

WHO ISN'T GETTING ENOUGH?

Thanks to a rolling government survey known as the National Diet and Nutrition Survey, we now have quite a good idea of who in the UK population is falling short on vitamins and minerals. The survey is a large-scale snapshot of exactly what people have bought and eaten over the previous four days, allowing for the calculation of actual vitamin and mineral intakes versus RNI recommendations.

On the surface, things look reasonably fine, with the *average* intake of most nutrients being adequate. However, dig deeper and this survey reveals quite large numbers of people who don't even consume the 'lower Reference Nutrient Intake' (or LRNI), defined as the daily amount that would be insufficient for 97% of people in a group.

Most notably, it is women and teenagers (and particularly teenage girls) who are most likely not to achieve LRNI amounts of nutrients, putting them at high risk of either being deficient or developing a deficiency. To pluck just two examples from the 2008/9–2010/11 survey, a fifth of girls aged between 11 and 18 and around one in eight women consume too little riboflavin (vitamin B2), and around a fifth of teenage girls and a tenth of teenage boys get insufficient zinc.

In fact, virtually anybody can become marginally short of nutrients if they don't eat a healthy or varied-enough diet. Over the next few chapters we'll help you decide which, if any, nutrients you're most likely to require topping up, and which would be the best supplement to buy if you decide to take one.

2

CHOOSING AND USING SUPPLEMENTS

WHO TAKES SUPPLEMENTS?

Research by the Food Standards Agency (FSA) in 2008 found that nearly a third of people in the UK take some vitamin, mineral or dietary supplement on most days, and about 15% report having taken a 'high dose' supplement in the last 12 months. Older people tend to be the biggest supplement consumers, according to National Diet and Nutrition Survey data, with 37% of over 65s, versus 25% of the adult population as a whole, reporting that they popped a pill in the last four days.

Data also suggests that women are more likely than men to take supplements, and that people in poorer health are also more likely to take them. Just over half of households with children (52%) say they give them to their offspring.

Market data shows that the two most popular supplement categories are multivitamins and fish oils. Products that target joint health also take a big slice of the market, accounting for 36% of sales. Supplements for the heart, bones and immune system are also very popular.

WHO NEEDS THEM?

Whether you could benefit from a supplement will depend on your personal circumstances. The information in this book, together with an honest appraisal of your diet (see page 8 for information on food groups to include) will give you a better idea. Certain people should definitely take a vitamin supplement, however – here are some specific recommendations from the UK Department of Health:

- Women trying to conceive and women in the first 12 weeks of their pregnancy should take folic acid, which reduces the chance that the baby will have a neural tube defect such as spina bifida.
- People aged 65 and over need to take vitamin D supplements.
- People with darker skin and people who are not exposed to much sun also need to take vitamin D supplements.
- All children aged six months to five years should be given a supplement containing vitamins A, C and D.

HOW ARE SUPPLEMENTS REGULATED?

If you take a supplement, you'll obviously want to know that it's safe and effective, and in theory there are enough safeguards in place to make this so. For example, EU Food Supplements legislation – a specific sub-branch of food law – specifies the vitamins and minerals and their chemical form that can be allowed in a supplement, and if a vitamin or mineral doesn't appear on the approved list it shouldn't be present in a product. The approved list contains all the vitamins and minerals that have designated RDAs (listed on page 6), plus boron, silicon, chloride, fluoride and sodium.

When it comes to herbal supplements, a drive towards tighter regulations means that many, such as echinacea or St John's wort, are now licensed under medicines legislation as 'registered traditional herbal medicines', which means they must pass strict safety and quality standards.

However, there are still many popular products (glucosamine, fish oils and coenzyme Q10, for example) that are not vitamins, minerals or licensed herbs. Falling under food and food supplements law they should have no medicinal effect, but can still influence certain bodily functions or systems. Therefore it pays to make sure you are only taking correctly formulated supplements from reputable sources.

Points to check when buying supplements:

- Is the company producing supplements to the highest quality standards in a plant that operates good manufacturing practice (GMP)? Any reputable company should be happy to immediately confirm this.
- Are vitamin and mineral levels present in non-toxic amounts? (See page 19 for information on safe upper levels.)
- Are 'miracle' claims being made for the supplement? This is a sure sign that the manufacturer may care less for your safety than about profits (see 'What Manufacturers Can and Can't Say', below).
- If it's a herbal product, is it a registered traditional herbal medicine (look for the THR trademark) or licensed medicine (with the letters PL and a nine-digit code listed on the label)? If not, you may need to be particularly careful as to the source and reputation of the product as unlicensed herbal supplements occasionally have been found to contain banned or toxic substances.

WHAT MANUFACTURERS CAN AND CAN'T SAY

Food supplement companies should not be making claims that their product treats or cures conditions (these are medical claims). However, they can claim to maintain a function. So whilst a calcium and vitamin D product couldn't claim to 'help prevent osteoporosis', it *would* be able to say 'helps maintain bone'. EU legislation controls the use of nutrition and health claims, and what can and can't be said is constantly being assessed and updated. It's best not to trust a supplement that makes obviously illegal or outrageous claims.

A TOUR ROUND A LABEL

The supplement label must carry various key pieces of information, including an ingredients box, a lot number and a best before date. Although labels can vary quite a lot in their precise layout, the following is a typical example.

VITALITY VITS B COMPLEX 90 TABLETS

Vitality Vits B Complex contains a selection of B vitamins that help to release the energy from your food. Vitality Vits B Complex can help to maintain your normal energy levels (1)

Ingredients: Microcrystalline Cellulose, Dicalcium Phosphate, Nicotinamide, Calcium Pantothenate, Silicon Dioxide, Magnesium Stearate, Croscarmellose Sodium, Pyridoxine, Hydrochloride, Riboflavin, Thiamine Mononitrate, Folic Acid, Biotin, Cyanocobalamin (2)

Vitamin food supplement. Food supplements should not be used as a substitute for a varied diet (3)

Suitable for vegetarians and vegans. Gluten free (4)

Directions: Take one or two tablets daily. Swallow whole with water or a cold drink (5)

Nutrition Information:

	Average per tablet	% RDA (6)
Vitamin B1	1.1mg	100
Vitamin B2	1.4mg	100
Niacin	16mg NE	100
Vitamin B6	400µg	100
Folic acid	2.5µg	200
Vitamin B12	5µg	200
Biotin	400µg	100
Pantothenic acid	6mg	100

Keep out of the reach of children. Store tightly closed in a cool, dry place (7)

LOT / BATCH NUMBER: 114399
BEST BEFORE END: Sep 16 (8)

Vitality Vitamins Ltd, Any Street, Any Town, UK (9)

(1) An example of an approved nutrition claim. As this is a food supplement, a claim like 'relieves fatigue' would not be allowed and could suggest a company prepared to flout the law in other areas too.

(2) All ingredients must be listed in descending weight order. This includes active and non-active ingredients (also known as excipients, used to fashion the supplement into tablet or capsule form), and it may not be immediately obvious which are active ingredients and which are excipients.

(3) All food supplements must define themselves as such somewhere on the packaging. Products must also include a statement explaining that supplements are not a substitute for a balanced diet.

(4) Whilst all the ingredients must be fully approved and safe, not all supplements will be suitable if you are vegetarian or have allergies. For example, stearic acid (a common excipient) can be from either an animal or a vegetable source.

(5) Do take care to follow the directions. Some products need to be taken with a main meal for full efficacy, for example.

(6) The percentage of the Recommended Daily Allowance provided by a unit dose of the supplement must be clearly shown. This is your opportunity to compare the potency of different products. In many cases though, for example with fish oils, probiotics or herbal supplements, there is no RDA.

(7) All products must carry a warning that supplements should be kept out of the reach of children. Supplements

should generally be kept in a cool, dry place in the original container, but check for any specific instructions.

(8) All products must bear a lot or batch number for full trace-ability, and a Best Before date. Products may lose potency after the Best Before date.

(9) The manufacturer's or distributor's name and address are required to appear on the label.

SAFE UPPER LEVELS

Obviously it's possible to have too much of a good thing, and if you're taking vitamins and minerals you need to be sure you aren't getting too high a dose. In 2003, the UK's Expert Group on Vitamins and Minerals (EVM) – an independent expert advisory committee – published an extensive review of the safe intakes of vitamins and minerals, and reputable manu-facturers will stick to these (shown in the table below).

Eight vitamins and minerals were given designated Safe Upper Levels (SULs), whilst several more were given Guidance Levels (meaning there wasn't strong enough evidence to determine a SUL, or no adverse effect of the nutrient was identified). SULs or GLs reflect the doses of vitamins and minerals that most people can 'take daily on a life-long basis, without medical supervision in reasonable safety'.

In many cases these levels will be a lot higher than you'll usually come across, but it is worth checking your dosages care-fully (particularly if you're taking more than one supplement) to make sure they don't breach these guidelines. At the moment there aren't any laws on the maximum (or indeed minimum) amount of vitamins or minerals allowed in supplements, and although Europe-wide figures known as Tolerable Upper Levels are being pulled together as a basis for future legislation, it's a slow process.

VITAMIN OR MINERAL	SAFE UPPER LEVEL (SUL) OR GUIDANCE LEVEL (GL)
Vitamin A	1500µg (GL) – 7mg if taken as beta carotene
Thiamin (B1)	100mg (GL)
Riboflavin (B2)	40mg (GL)
Niacin (B3)	500mg (GL)
Pantothenic acid (B5)	200mg (GL)
Vitamin B6	10mg (SUL)
Biotin (also known as B7)	900µg (GL)
Folic acid (also known as B9)	1000µg (GL)
Vitamin B12	2000µg (GL)
Vitamin C	1000mg (GL)
Vitamin D	25µg (GL)
Vitamin E	540mg (SUL)
Vitamin K	1000µg (GL)
Potassium	3700mg (GL)
Calcium	1500mg (GL)
Phosphorus	250mg (GL)
Magnesium	400mg (GL)
Iron	17mg (GL)

VITAMIN OR MINERAL	SAFE UPPER LEVEL (SUL) OR GUIDANCE LEVEL (GL)
Zinc	25mg (SUL)
Copper	10mg (SUL)
Manganese	4mg (GL)
Selenium	350µg (SUL)
Molybdenum	200µg (GL)
Chromium	10mg (GL)
Iodine	500µg (GL)

TABLET, CAPSULE OR LIQUID?

CAPSULES

PROS: Can be easier to swallow than equivalent tablet formulations and may contain fewer non-active ingredients.
CONS: Not always suitable for vegetarians – they may contain gelatin.

TABLETS

PROS: Tend to be less expensive than comparable capsules.
CONS: Not always easy to swallow, depending on size and shape.

CHEWABLE OR EFFERVESCENT

PROS: Good if you can't swallow tablets or capsules.
CONS: Contain sugar and/or sweeteners.

LIQUID
PROS: Good if you struggle with swallowing tablets, and can be easier to get a higher dose (of fish oils for example).
CONS: Messy, not very portable.

TIMED-RELEASE FORMULATIONS
PROS: 'Trickle' water-soluble vitamins (B and C) into the system, keeping levels higher for longer.
CONS: More expensive. The benefits of time-released vitamins aren't proven either.

DOES TIMING MATTER?

What time of day should you take vitamins? Many people think it should be in the morning, but timing is, on the whole, unimportant. What matters more is establishing a daily routine so that you don't forget your vitamins one day and then take too many the next. Unless the label specifically states otherwise, it is best to take supplements with a meal, as components of the meal, such as fat, will help the vitamins and minerals to be absorbed by the body better.

3

THE BIG THREE: MULTIVITAMINS, FISH OILS AND GLUCOSAMINE

Market surveys consistently place multivitamins and fish oils as top of the UK supplement bestsellers list, and glucosamine (for joints) as a popular third – perhaps reflecting the fact that we are becoming an increasingly ageing population. Given these are such widely used supplements, we've devoted a separate chapter to them. What are their purported benefits? Who might need them? And which should you pick from the wide variety of formulations available?

MULTIVITAMINS

Not surprisingly, multivitamins are one of the most popular types of supplements to take, as they are rightly perceived as good all-rounders, providing basic nutritional insurance. Most 'multivitamins' also include a wide range of minerals.

Who might need multivitamins?

Harvard University's School of Public Health – a world-renowned authority in health and wellness – recommends that all adults consume a daily multivitamin. Even supplement-sceptic experts will acknowledge that a multivitamin can help plug the gaps at times when you aren't eating well or are on a restricted diet. Other times or reasons you might want to take a multivitamin include: when you're short on sleep or highly stressed, if you're a breast-feeding mother, a smoker, or are drinking too much alcohol.

What's the benefit?

If you take a multivitamin when you don't happen to need one you won't notice any effect. However, if by taking one you correct one or more nutritional deficiencies, the benefits could include enhanced energy levels and a better physical response to stress, better memory and concentration, and improved immune-system response (i.e. being less prone to infections).

Tips on choosing and using

- Look for a comprehensive A–Z-style supplement that has 100% of the RDA for most nutrients. It's OK if levels are higher as long as they don't exceed the Safe Upper Levels on page 20.

- Nutrients that won't be present at RDA levels, no matter how good the multivitamin is, include calcium and magnesium, as these are simply too bulky to include in these levels in a multivitamin. However, it's reasonable to expect a multi to contain 20–25% of these two minerals' RDAs (unless you're taking then separately).

- Before the menopause, a women's multi should ideally contain 400 micrograms of folic acid, which helps make and maintain new cells and which can reduce the incidence of neural tube birth defects, such as spina bifida, should she fall pregnant. If it doesn't, consider topping up with an extra 200 micrograms of folic acid.

- Younger women should also look for a multivitamin with the full RDA (14mg) of iron to replace the iron lost during menstruation. Men and postmenopausal women are OK with multis that contain less or no iron.

- If you are a pregnant woman you may want to look for a product that's specially formulated for pregnancy, as the UK government advises that pregnant women should not take vitamin A, on the basis that too much may harm the foetus. However, if you didn't realise you were pregnant and have been taking a standard multivitamin that contains 800 micrograms (the RDA) of vitamin A, don't panic. It's only much higher vitamin A levels (such as the 25,000 micrograms in a portion of calves' liver) that are of particular worry. In short, government advice for pregnant women to avoid liver is very valid; advice not to take just 800 micrograms of vitamin A in the form of a daily supplement is less so.

- If you're over 65, or are a pregnant or breast-feeding woman, look for a multi that contains 10 micrograms of vitamin D (200% of the RDA), or else take some extra vitamin D separately to get up to this level.

- If you're on blood-thinning drugs and decide to start taking multivitamins, you may need one that doesn't contain vitamin K, as the vitamin aids blood clotting. You should check with your GP or consultant to be sure.

- It is always best to take multivitamins with a meal, as some components in a multivitamin – such as zinc, for example – may cause nausea if taken on an empty stomach.

Safety

Can multivitamins sometimes do harm? A highly publicised study in the *Annals of Internal Medicine* in 2011 seemed to suggest so, as it correlated multivitamin use with a higher risk of dying in women aged over 55. However, the study is regarded by experts as fatally flawed, as it did not exclude individuals who were already ill, and did not take into account that women might have started taking supplements for the very reason that their health had started to deteriorate. On balance, the overwhelming evidence is that multivitamins are perfectly safe.

SPECIALIST MULTIVITAMINS

In essence there are two categories of more specialist multivitamins – those that are A–Z style but formulated for particular age groups or life stages, and those, such as B complex and antioxidant supplements, that can still be considered 'multis' but have a smaller sub-range of vitamins, often (but not always) in higher doses.

Choosing a supplement that's especially formulated for your needs (50s, pregnancy, and so on) has its advantages, but it may work out more expensive than a cheaper generic type, and is by no means essential if you follow the basic guidelines above on what to choose.

With specialist multis of the antioxidant/B complex type, each individual product must be taken on its merits, though there's little logical reason you would take these in place of an A–Z multivitamin (and if you're taking them in addition you may be doubling up in places you don't need to). With antioxidants specifically, it's worth being particularly careful as some may be actually harmful in certain circumstances, perhaps even at doses that don't exceed the Safe Upper Level (see 'The Lowdown on Antioxidants', page 57).

FISH OILS

Since spoonfuls of cod liver oil were poured down the throats of wartime toddlers, the consumption of fish oil, rich in omega-3 oils, has remained a strong tradition in Britain. 'Fish oil' encompasses two main categories of product: cod liver oils (obtained, as the name suggests, from the liver of this white fish) and fish oil concentrates obtained from the flesh of oily fish such as salmon or sardines. Both are rich in the omega-3 oils EPA and DHA (eicosapentaenoic acid and docosohexaenoic acid), but cod liver oil also contain vitamins A and D. A third type of omega-3-rich fish oil, known as krill oil, comes from small crustaceans.

Who might need fish oils?

In theory, people who eat oily fish regularly (at least one meal a week) should not need to take fish oils. However, if you don't eat oily fish regularly and don't think you'll be changing your habits any time soon (three-quarters of Britons don't eat oily fish at all), a supplement offers a viable alternative. Women of childbearing age who already eat two portions of oily fish a week but would like more omega-3 also need to use supplements to top up, because of contaminant concerns with the whole fish.

What's the benefit?

Known primarily for their healthy heart benefits, the omega-3s in oily fish help keep blood flowing freely round blood vessels. More particularly, they reduce blood 'stickiness', and its tendency to clot, by helping to lower levels of blood fats called triglycerides. There's also evidence that omega-3s may help to prevent arrhythmias (irregular heartbeats) and to lower blood pressure.

How this translates into real-life effects is less clear, however, with two large reviews in 2012 showing little evidence that omega-3 supplements reduced cardiovascular risk. The bottom line seems to be that it is always best to eat a healthy, Mediterranean-style diet rich in oily fish rather than rely on supplements. But the situation is also complicated by the fact that modern heart medications may obscure the benefits of fish oil in clinical trials. However, one valuable thing that fish oil supplements can do is to make it less likely a person will die if they do experience a heart attack or stroke.

Fish oils – or the omega-3s in them – may also help give some relief in inflammatory joint conditions, in particular rheumatoid arthritis. This type of arthritis is an autoimmune disorder, and omega-3s seem to work in these conditions by suppressing the immune response that causes inflammation and pain. Psoriasis, eczema and asthma are other autoimmune conditions that may benefit from fish oils for the same reason.

Studies show that fish oils are also helpful for pregnant women, and may reduce the risk of having a preterm birth. The omega-3s they provide are essential to the unborn child's development, particularly in the last three months of pregnancy, when an infant's IQ and immune functions appear to be programmed.

Depression and Alzheimer's are two other conditions where fish oils have purported benefits, though the evidence here is very mixed.

Tips on choosing and using
- Check the EPA/DHA content – if you never eat oily fish you should choose a supplement that provides around 450mg of these two combined a day (this is about equal to one 140g portion of oily fish a week).

- People who have already had a heart attack may need a higher amount of 1000mg EPA/DHA a day, though this increased recommendation is being deleted from NICE (National Institute of Health and Care Excellence) guidelines (fish oils are now deemed less important with the advent of effective heart medications).
- To reduce pain and inflammation in rheumatoid arthritis you may need up to 3000mg of EPA and DHA a day.
- If you have been diagnosed with high levels of triglycerides, you may need a more concentrated form of omega-3 still, only available on prescription. Speak to your GP or consultant.
- Cod liver oil supplements are ideal if you'd also like a top-up of vitamins A and D. Cod liver oil can be a good choice for the over 65s in particular, as they need at least 10 micrograms of supplemental vitamin D per day.
- Don't take cod liver oil in pregnancy, as too much vitamin A can be harmful to the baby. Pregnant women who aren't eating much oily fish should look for an omega-3 supplement that is free of vitamin A but also has a higher ratio of DHA to EPA, as DHA is the omega-3 fat most strongly linked with foetal development.
- Want to go straight to the most potent omega-3 supplement on the shelf? This will almost always be a liquid supplement, on the basis that you can fit more on a spoon than you can in a capsule.
- Keep fish oils somewhere cool and dark (in the fridge or in a paper bag for liquids). Omega-3s are chemically sensitive oils that break down with heat and light.
- Take fish oils with a main meal to minimise 'fishy burps'.

Safety

Fish oil supplements have come under scrutiny a few times in the last 15 years, with some products exceeding recommended levels of PCBs (Polychlorinated biphenyls) and dioxins linked to cancer. Given that many people who are taking fish oil supplements may be doing do so for the very reason that they want to avoid the toxins present in oily fish, this seems rather alarming. Reassuringly though, the legal maximums for PCBs/dioxins in fish oils are very stringent, so that on the whole it's much safer in terms of dioxin/PCB levels to consume supplemental fish oil than to eat fish, even when there are occasional breaches. However, always choose a reputable manufacturer, and don't be afraid to ask to see a certificate of analysis indicating the purity level.

Contrary to previous thinking, fish oil, even in relatively high doses, probably doesn't cause significant excessive bleeding – should you cut yourself, for example. If you are taking warfarin or a similar anticoagulant, you should of course talk to your GP and continue to be monitored as usual.

Taking more than 3g of omega-3 supplements daily may worsen glucose control in people with diabetes.

Headlines linking high blood levels of omega-3 fatty acids with aggressive prostate cancer shouldn't concern male consumers of fish oil as the research in question did not actually measure fish oil intake and high omega-3 blood levels may be the result of cancer not the cause of it. Other studies show oily fish consumption to be linked with lower prostate cancer risk.

FISH VS FISH OIL SUPPLEMENTS

When you're weighing up oily fish versus supplements, 450mg of fish oil is equivalent to one 140g oily fish portion a week, 1000mg a day is equivalent to two to three oily fish portions a week, and 3000mg is equivalent to one oily fish portion a day. Only a certain amount of omega-3 should be obtained through eating whole fish, though, because of concerns over PCB/dioxin toxins. The UK Food Standards Agency says up to four oily fish portions a week is safe for males, but girls and women who are pregnant or could become pregnant (or who are breast-feeding), should have no more than two portions a week. If you want to routinely consume omega-3 above the fish consumption levels that are safe for you, you should do it with supplements.

EVENING PRIMROSE: ANOTHER SPECIAL OIL?

Evening primrose oil used to be a very popular supplement, but its popularity seems to have waned in recent times. One reason may be that it contains omega-6 fats, which have fallen out of favour over the last few years as we now know we generally eat too much of them in proportion to omega-3s. However, evening primrose oil is unusual in containing 10% gamma-linolenic acid (GLA), which is one of the few omega-6 fats that is anti-inflammatory, rather than pro-inflammatory.

Evidence suggests that evening primrose oil is not as good a treatment for eczema as once thought, and the evidence that it can help with menopausal and premenstrual symptoms is also very weak. Some women still swear by it for easing cyclical breast pains, though, and another area where it could help is in easing nerve pain in people with damage to nerves due to diabetes complications. People with allergies can also have lower levels of GLA in their blood and may want to top up with a supplement.

If you take a high dose of evening primrose oil it's a good idea to cut down a bit on other omega-6-rich plant oil sources, like corn oil, in your diet.

GLUCOSAMINE

A supplement that has become hugely popular in recent years, glucosamine is a naturally occurring building block of cartilage – the tough, flexible tissue that covers and protects the surface of joints.

Who might need glucosamine?

Given that collagen levels tend to fall as we age, it is older people with worn joints who would theoretically be the most likely to benefit from a glucosamine supplement. Amongst the many thousands of loyal users of glucosamine are also athletes and sports people, particularly those trying to ward off damage to knee cartilage.

What's the benefit?

Glucosamine is widely thought of as beneficial for people with osteoarthritis – the wear-and-tear type of arthritis associated with ageing. Many GPs used to advocate it as a low-risk alternative to non-steroidal anti-inflammatory drugs for joint pain, but with many more clinical studies now completed, the picture has become more complicated. Glucosamine studies have shown varying results of effectiveness and can be confusing to decipher.

On the positive side, several studies, particularly the earlier ones, show glucosamine as having better efficacy than placebos, and equal effectiveness to ibuprofen, in terms of benefits such as reducing the pain and stiffness of osteoarthritis. In addition, unlike conventional treatments, one three-year study of over 200 people found glucosamine treatment prevented progressive damage to the knee joint (this was demonstrated through X-rays). Another large study found similar results, whilst a follow-up analysis, done five years later, found suggestive evidence that use of glucosamine reduced the need for knee-replacement surgery.

However, a number of studies have been less promising, with glucosamine administration resulting in little meaningful improvement in symptoms. One study involving 147 women with osteoarthritis found glucosamine to be only as effective as home exercises over an 18-month period, whilst a systematic review of ten trials involving nearly 4000 patients with osteoarthritis of hip or knee, found that glucosamine, alone or with chondroitin, did not improve pain.

One possibility, as suggested by a study in the *New England Journal of Medicine*, is that the effectiveness of glucosamine may depend on the severity of arthritis pain, with those experiencing the most discomfort feeling the biggest benefit.

Additionally, as with all research – and a great deal has been carried out on glucosamine – the quality of studies varies and conclusions can be difficult to draw. Osteoarthritis is also a notoriously tricky condition to assess, with symptoms that wax and wane.

Official guidance from the National Institute of Health and Care Excellence (NICE) is that doctors should not prescribe glucosamine for osteoarthritis for cost-effectiveness reasons. However it advises patients aiming to self-manage the condition with glucosamine that they could experience mild to moderate pain reduction, and should monitor symptoms before starting glucosamine and again three months afterwards. Exercising and weight management should ideally be teamed with supplement self-help.

If you're giving it a go, these pointers will help you get the best out of glucosamine:

Tips on choosing and using
- Look for either glucosamine hydrochloride or glucosamine sulphate. There is some dispute over which chemical form

of glucosamine is best, but one study provided evidence that these two are equally effective.

- The useful dose is 1500mg a day, and there is some evidence that taking it all in one go, rather than 500mg three times a day, is better.
- If you're vegetarian or have a shellfish allergy, look for glucosamine supplements that are produced (sustainably) from corn. Many products on the market are sourced from mollusc shells.
- Supplements that combine glucosamine with chondroitin – another major component of cartilage and other connective tissue – may be better than glucosamine alone, according to animal studies. But additional ingredients should not dilute the glucosamine dose, which should still be 1500mg a day.

Safety

Glucosamine has an extremely good safety record with no known side effects. People with shellfish allergies will need to avoid marine-sourced glucosamine though.

WHAT ARE THOSE OTHER THINGS IN MY GLUCOSAMINE SUPPLEMENT?

As well, or instead of, chondroitin (see above), some glucosamine supplements may also contain *bromelain*, which occurs naturally in fresh pineapple. Higher levels of bromelain than are found in food can have a beneficial effect on reducing inflammation from infection and injury, and the German Commission E, which determines which herbs can be safely prescribed in Germany, has approved bromelain to treat swelling and inflammation after surgery.

Another candidate you could find vying for a place in your joint supplement is *MSM*, or *methyl sulfonyl methane* – a natural component of foods, which supplies the sulphur needed in the maintenance of connective tissue. Again, there are some trials that show a benefit in osteo-arthritis, but so far there's not enough detailed evidence to convincingly determine whether MSM is useful or not.

In the end it may be best to try a few glucosamine-based joint supplements with different adjunct ingredients to see what combination works for you.

4

AN A–Z OF VITAMINS AND MINERALS

VITAMINS

VITAMIN A

RDA: 800μg; *Safe Upper Level*: 1500μg

Food sources
Liver is an astonishingly rich source of vitamin A, whilst eggs, fortified breakfast cereals, full-fat dairy products and oily fish such as herrings and kippers contain much less. Other good sources are orange/red and deep green vegetables, such as carrots, red peppers and spinach, which contain the precursor form of vitamin A called beta carotene (see page 38). Beta carotene has antioxidant properties in its own right, but is also converted into vitamin A as the body requires.

What it does
Vitamin A is needed for our immune defences, being vital for the health of protective mucous surfaces that keep germs out of the respiratory tract, vagina and gut. Vitamin A is also needed for the skin to maintain its protective oil layer, which in turn may help prevent spots and infection. The vitamin is important for eyesight and a lack of it continues to be the leading cause of preventable blindness in children, which is

tragically common in areas of the world where vitamin A intake is extremely low.

BETA CAROTENE:
THE PLANT SOURCE OF VITAMIN A

The 'ready to use' form of vitamin A (called retinol) is only found in animal-source foods. But the beta carotene in orange/red or deep green fruit and vegetables can be converted into retinol as the body requires, so vegetarians should have no problem achieving their intake of the vitamin. In fact, just one carrot has enough beta carotene to provide the RDA.

But beta carotene doesn't only act as a vitamin A precursor – it also acts as an antioxidant, mopping up the free radicals that can damage cells. Evidence suggests that getting plentiful beta carotene from fruit and vegetables is safe, and may reduce your risk of heart disease, cancer and diabetes, but high doses of beta carotene in supplement form haven't proved effective against these diseases, and may even do some harm in certain scenarios. When taken by smokers, for example, 20mg–30mg of beta carotene actually increases the risk of lung cancer by about 24%, a 2008 review of research in the journal *Cancer* concluded.

The bottom line seems to be that whilst beta carotene in food is safe and beneficial, high doses of beta carotene in supplement form stop being helpful and may even do some harm. That's why the Safe Upper Level is a maximum dose of 7mg of beta carotene in supplement form – which is no more than the amount that a healthy diet can supply. And if you're a smoker, don't take beta carotene supplements at all.

Who might need a top-up?

Men and boys are those who are most likely to consume quite low levels of vitamin A. You won't be short if you eat your 5-a-day and include a variety of colourful fruits and vegetables.

Supplement tips

- Cod liver oil and multivitamins are the two best ways to get vitamin A in supplement form.
- 800 micrograms (100% of the RDA) would be a typical useful dose in a multivitamin, though it doesn't necessarily mean it's a poor supplement if it has less – check how much there is of everything else.

Caution!

High levels of vitamin A can harm the foetus, so pregnant women should look for a multivitamin without it.

VITAMIN B1 (THIAMIN)

RDA: 1.1mg; *Safe Upper Level*: 100mg

Food sources

Potatoes, peas and nuts are good sources, though it is widespread in lots of foods.

What it does

Vitamin B1 plays a crucial role in the biochemical pathway known as the Krebs cycle, which converts the energy bound in carbohydrates, fats and proteins into a useable form. Without it, it would be impossible for the billions of cells in our bodies to make the energy we need to live. The vitamin also helps in the functioning of the nervous system and in the transmission of nerve impulses.

Who might need a top-up?

The average diet, even if not optimal, generally provides enough vitamin B1 and there are no specific 'at risk' groups, nor any indication of deficiency, in the UK population. Pregnant and lactating women have higher needs, but these are usually covered by a healthy diet.

Supplement tips

It makes sense that a multivitamin would contain 100% of the RDA, for the sake of completeness (and because vitamins tend to work in combination with each other). But it's one of the nutrients in a supplement that you're probably least likely to need.

VITAMIN B2 (RIBOFLAVIN)

RDA: 1.4mg; *Safe Upper Level*: 40mg

Food sources

Dairy products are amongst the best sources of riboflavin, but it is also found in whole grains and fortified cereals, and there is some in meat and fish.

What it does

Like thiamin and several other B vitamins, riboflavin helps to release energy from the carbohydrates, proteins and fats that we eat. The vitamin also plays an important role in the production and repair of body tissues. It is essential for healthy hair, skin and nails.

Who might need a top-up?

Dietary and Nutrition Survey statistics suggest a fifth of girls aged 11 to 18 and about one in eight women consume low levels of vitamin B2, which could be corrected by consuming an extra glass of milk or a multivitamin daily. Pregnant and breast-feeding women may particularly need to watch their intake, as they require 30–50% higher amounts than at other times.

Supplement tips
A good all-round multivitamin should contain 100% of the RDA of riboflavin.

Caution!
Too much vitamin B2 may not harm you, but it may give you alarmingly yellow wee! The vitamin is a vibrant yellow colour and the excess that is excreted means your urine can take on this hue.

VITAMIN B3 (NIACIN)
RDA: 16mg; *Safe Upper Level*: up to 500mg

Food sources
Meat, oily fish, poultry, bread, potatoes and breakfast cereals. Niacin can also be synthesised from tryptophan (an essential amino acid in protein foods).

What it does
Niacin helps form NAD (nicotinamide adenine dinucleotide) and NADP (nicotinamide adenine dinucleotide phosphate), which are vital facilitators in the release of energy. Niacin is also vital to maintain a healthy nervous and digestive system and is essential for normal growth and for healthy skin.

Who might need a top-up?
Whilst still a problem in some developing countries, niacin

deficiency is virtually unheard of in the typical UK diet, and so it's usually only included in multivitamins for the sake of completeness.

B COMPLEX VITAMINS AND STRESS

Most B vitamins are sold together as a complex, and they are often promoted to relieve stress. But according to evidence, how much does a B complex supplement help? If you happen to be particularly low in one or more B vitamins, probably quite a lot, as collectively they are important for a healthy nervous system. It doesn't mean, however, that taking mega doses of them will somehow make you super-resilient to physical or emotional stress, or fantastically more energised. That said, at least a couple of studies have found improvement in areas such as cognitive performance, dejected mood and work place stress when given higher than RDA amounts of B complex. Researchers conclude that the people who benefit in such trials will probably have been marginally deficient in B vitamins to start with, but also leave open the possibility that people who aren't conventionally deficient in Bs may get a little extra boost in by taking a higher dose.

The verdict: a good diet or just a modest top-up of B vitamins is probably all you need to make sure you're bolstered against stress, but there's always the possibility that a higher dose might have benefits for the highly stressed. Always keep to the Safe Upper Levels indicated on page 20 and you'll be OK.

Supplement tips
- A good multivitamin will usually contain 100% of the RDA of niacin, for the sake of completeness and because B vitamins work together.
- You may see 'NE' in brackets in the nutritional panel of a supplement that contains niacin. This stands for 'niacin equivalents' and reflects the fact that the vitamin can also be made from the amino acid tryptophan.

Caution!
High doses of one type of niacin – nicotinic acid – can cause unpleasant facial flushing. For this reason most supplements use the nicotinamide form of niacin, which is free from side effects, even in doses up to 500mg. But if you're taking several different supplements it's worth just checking that you're not taking more than 17mg of nicotinic acid in total.

PANTOTHENIC ACID (VITAMIN B5)
RDA: 6mg; *Safe Upper Level*: 200mg

Food sources
Pantothenic acid is widely found in all food groups (*pante* means 'everywhere' in Greek), and you'll get it in dairy, meat, cereals and veg.

What it does
Pantothenic acid works with other B vitamins in metabolising carbohydrates, proteins and fats. It also helps in the manufacture of antibodies, which are needed to fight infections.

Who might need a top-up?
Because of its widespread occurrence in food, pantothenic acid

is not generally measured in diet surveys, with the assumption that most of us get enough.

Supplement tips
It's unlikely that you'd need more than 100% of the RDA, so look for this amount in multivitamin formulations.

VITAMIN B6

RDA: 1.4mg; *Safe Upper Level*: 10mg

Food sources
Wholemeal bread, meat (especially liver and pork), fish, bananas, bran and fortified breakfast cereals. Most foods, though, provide some level of vitamin B6.

What it does
Another important member of the vitamin B complex, vitamin B6 (also known as pyridoxine) is needed for the metabolism of proteins in the body, and also helps the nervous system in a number of ways. It is required for the production of serotonin, a brain chemical affecting mood, behaviour and sleep patterns.

Along with vitamin B12 and folic acid, vitamin B6 also plays a role in maintaining low homocysteine levels in the blood. Studies have shown that elevated blood levels of homo-cysteine can be a risk factor for heart disease and stroke.

Who might need a top-up?
Because vitamin B6 is so widespread in food, most people get enough. There's some evidence that the contraceptive pill can deplete levels, however, so women who take this form of

CAN FOLIC ACID, B6 AND B12 STAVE OFF ALZHEIMER'S?

Researchers at Oxford University have found that in older people who have mild cognitive impairment and high homocysteine levels, high doses of vitamins B6, B12 and folic acid (B9) can significantly reduce brain shrinkage in areas of the brain associated with Alzheimer's. The researchers surmise that if caught early enough (and, to stress again, only in people who test positive for high homocysteine levels), these three B vitamins may slow the mental decline into Alzheimer's, though at this stage this is far from proven. The study used 800 micrograms of folic acid, 20mg of vitamin B6 and 500 micrograms of vitamin B12, but it's possible that lower levels might be as good too – we just don't know. For older people, with potential B12 absorption issues and mental decline already apparent, there's much more logic to higher doses than with younger people, but always check with a doctor before taking higher levels than the Safe Upper Level.

contraception may need to take particular care to ensure they get a good intake.

Supplements of vitamin B6 are sometimes recommended for helping with mood swings and irritability, and there is some scientific support for its use for mild symptoms of PMS (premenstrual syndrome). Pregnant women might also want to try a supplement of the vitamin to ease pregnancy sickness.

Supplement tips
- Look for a supplement with 100% of the RDA for general nutritional health.
- For premenstrual women, up to 10mg would be worth trying.

Caution!

Taking more than 200mg a day of vitamin B6 for a long time can lead to a loss of feeling in the arms and legs, known as peripheral neuropathy. Generally, the symptoms are reversible, so once you stop taking supplements the symptoms usually stop. However, in a few cases when people have taken large amounts of vitamin B6, especially for more than a few months, the effect has been irreversible. Taking doses of 10mg–200mg a day for short periods may not cause any harm, but Department of Health advice is not to take more than 10mg of vitamin B6 a day routinely in supplements, unless advised to by a doctor.

BIOTIN (ALSO KNOWN AS VITAMIN B7)
RDA: 50µg; *Safe Upper Level*: 900µg

Food sources
The richest sources of biotin are liver, kidney, eggs and soya beans. Meat, wholegrain cereals, wholemeal bread, milk and cheese are also good sources, but fruit and vegetables contain very little biotin.

What it does
Like many of the other B vitamins, biotin is involved in the metabolism of food components. It is of central importance in metabolising fats, and helps in making a supply of essential glucose when energy intakes are low. Biotin is also known to be important in maintaining healthy skin and hair.

Who might need a top-up?
Most people get enough biotin and deficiency is unknown in healthy adults eating a normal diet. However, a scaly skin condition can be induced by the bizarre (and unhealthy)

consumption of large amounts of raw egg whites, which contain a factor that binds biotin.

Supplement tips
Look for up to 100% of the RDA in a multivitamin or B complex.

FOLIC ACID (ALSO KNOWN AS VITAMIN B9)
RDA: 200µg; *Safe Upper Level*: 1000µg

Food sources
The vitamin is found in green leafy vegetables, pulses, orange juice, potatoes, yeast extract, liver and fortified breakfast cereals.

What it does
Folic acid (also known as folacin and folate) is a B vitamin needed for cell division, and, along with vitamin B12, for the production of healthy red blood cells. It is also crucial for the development of an unborn baby's spinal cord. It has been proven that supplementing with folic acid during pregnancy can markedly decrease the incidence of spina bifida.

There is some evidence that folic acid may help prevent precancerous cell changes, and low folic acid levels are associated with early stage abnormalities in the cervix, colon and lung.

In the area of emotional health, it is biochemically plausible that having an adequate level of folic acid could decrease the risk of depression, as the vitamin affects levels of serotonin and other neurotransmitters that are linked to mental health.

Folic acid, along with other B vitamins, also helps lower blood levels of homocysteine. Studies have found that people with high levels of homocysteine are more likely to have heart attacks and strokes, but, disappointingly, recent research has found that lowering homocysteine via vitamin supplements does not appear to reduce this risk much. For Alzheimer's disease, however, there may be more promise (see page 45).

Who might need a top-up?

All women of childbearing age who are planning to have a baby or who may become pregnant are advised to take a supplement containing 400 micrograms of folic acid every day. This should be continued through the first three months of pregnancy.

People on antidepressants might benefit from folic acid in a supplement, as there's a suggestion that mood-lifting medications may not work if people are short of this B vitamin.

Supplement tips

- It's generally best to take folic acid in conjunction with other B vitamins (such as vitamin B12 and vitamin B6) in a B complex or A–Z multivitamin.
- During the first three months of pregnancy, and whilst preparing for conception, a 400-microgram folic acid supplement is necessary (but, if you're already pregnant, not in a product that also contains vitamin A).
- 400 micrograms of folic acid a day is the correct amount for women of childbearing age.
- Men and postmenopausal women shouldn't routinely need more than 200 micrograms of folic acid (100% of the RDA) from a supplement – and it may not be wise to take more if you have had colon cancer or polyps (see below).

Caution!

Though getting a good intake of folic acid may reduce the risk of colon cancer, large amounts of folic acid could potentially fuel tumour progression in those who already have precancerous growths or cancer. This potential danger probably doesn't kick in until a dose of 10,000 micrograms a day, but if you are not a woman of childbearing age there would seem little benefit to routinely taking more than 100% of the RDA (200µg), in supplement form anyway. (An exception could be in cases of Alzheimer's – see page 45.) Intakes of 1000 micrograms or more of folic acid will also 'mask' a vitamin B12 deficiency, and thus delay its diagnosis and treatment.

VITAMIN B12

RDA 2.5µg; *Safe Upper Level*: 2000µg

Food sources
Meat, fish, dairy foods and eggs are all good vitamin B12 sources.

What it does
Vitamin B12 (also called cobalamin) works closely with folic acid, another B vitamin, in the production of new cells, in particular red blood cells. Vitamin B12 also helps in nervous function and is required for the health of the myelin sheath, a protective casing around nerve fibres that speeds up the passage of nerve transmissions. Recent studies have found that consuming adequate amounts of B12 and other B vitamins such as folate (folic acid) and B6 is crucial in keeping the ageing brain healthy.

Who might need a top-up?
Vegetarians, and particularly vegans (who also avoid eggs and dairy products as well as meat and fish), need to get vitamin B12 from fortified foods or supplements as the vitamin is only found in animal food sources. Over 50s are also likely to benefit from a supplement, as getting B12 from food involves

a complex chemical process that can become harder with age: ageing may mean we do not produce enough stomach acid for it to happen efficiently.

Supplements provide a more easily absorbed form of vitamin B12 than that available in food sources, which is why the Institute of Medicine (which devises recommended nutrient intakes for the US and Canadian governments) advises people over 50 to get at least some of their B12 from supplements and/or fortified foods.

Supplement tips
- Look for formulations that contain 2.5 micrograms (100% of the RDA) as a minimum.
- Higher levels – e.g. 10µg–25µg – might be a good idea if you are older, as vitamin B12 is a safe vitamin, even in doses up to 1000µg–2000µg daily.

WHEN A B12 SUPPLEMENT ISN'T ENOUGH

No matter how much vitamin B12 you consume, it won't solve a deficiency if you're unlucky enough to have a complete lack of 'intrinsic factor'. This substance is a vital protein, produced by the stomach lining, which must combine with vitamin B12 in the gut in order for the B12 to be absorbed. In rare cases an individual's production of intrinsic factor can fall so low as to make any absorption of vitamin B12 virtually impossible, leading to the condition known as pernicious (megaloblastic) anaemia. Only around 2% of people will be affected by pernicious anaemia in their lifetime, but if you are (symptoms include extreme fatigue, dementia, disorientation, and weakness in the limbs), the only way to cure it is with vitamin B12 injections.

VITAMIN C

RDA: 80mg; *Safe Upper Level*: 1000mg

Food sources
Fruit and veg, and in particular citrus fruits, peppers, strawberries, blackcurrants and leafy green veg such as watercress.

What it does
Vitamin C (also called ascorbic acid) helps the body resist infection and helps maintain the health of our skin, gums and blood vessels. The vitamin is essential for the action of white blood cells that scavenge bacteria and viruses, and it is also an antioxidant that helps to protect the body's cells from attack by highly reactive molecules called free radicals.

Who might need a top-up?
Most diets, apart from those that are particularly inadequate, provide enough vitamin C, and average intake in the UK is around 200mg per day. That said, surveys show that around 1 in 100 adults, and up to 1 in 50 over 65s, may not be getting enough to avoid deficiency symptoms such as lowered immunity to infections and skin and gum problems. This can be easily remedied by consuming more fruit and veg.

Smokers use up more vitamin C than non smokers (though the RDA of 80mg should still be enough for them), and studies indicate that people who are physically stressed could also benefit from higher levels to prevent colds (see below).

Supplement tips
- 100% of the RDA in an A–Z multivitamin is the maximum amount of vitamin C most people will need, but if you're very physically active taking 200mg could be useful.

- If you want to take a higher dose of 1000mg, bear in mind that ascorbic acid can sometimes upset sensitive stomachs. If you are affected, try swapping to a non-acidic version such as calcium ascorbate (e.g. Ester C).

Caution!

Recent research indicates that at very high levels, vitamin C may turn from being a beneficial antioxidant into a potentially harmful pro-oxidant, which is a good reason to stick to a dose of no more than 1000mg a day. Mega doses of vitamin C (several grams a day) can cause nausea, diarrhoea and stomach cramps. And high doses can also cause rises in the blood sugar levels of people with diabetes. Too much vitamin C can also be dangerous for people with genetic conditions that cause an excessive build-up of iron in their body, such as haemochromatosis.

DOES VITAMIN C HELP COLDS?

Whether vitamin C can cure or prevent colds has been a matter of debate for some 60 years. The most respected review of the available research evidence was published by the Cochrane Library in 2007. It showed evidence that vitamin C supplementation with at least 200mg per day is beneficial in preventing colds in people undergoing physical stress, such as marathon runners and skiers. Vitamin C supplementation helped to stave off infection, and in fact halved their risk of getting a cold. For the majority of people, outside this group, it showed no great benefit in preventing colds. However, it found that higher doses of vitamin C (1000mg per day) reduced the duration of colds by 8% in adults and 13% in children (at least half a day).

VITAMIN D

RDA: 5µg; *Safe Upper Level*: 25µg

Food sources

Oily fish such as salmon, sardines and pilchards. Eggs, fortified breakfast cereals and full-fat dairy products also supply some vitamin D. The vitamin is also made in the skin by the action of sunlight.

What it does

Vitamin D works with calcium to keep bones strong, and there's evidence it can also prevent falls in the elderly – probably by helping to keep muscles strong. There are hints from research that it may also reduce the risk of heart disease, multiple sclerosis, diabetes, depression and some cancers. Lower levels of vitamin D are associated with obesity too. It's true that nearly all of this research has been laboratory or observational studies, rather than the large, long-term clinical trials that can prove cause and effect, but most vitamin D researchers agree there is a strong case that the vitamin is very important for health, beyond just its bone-strengthening effects.

Who might need a top-up?

According to the government's National Diet and Nutrition Survey, low blood levels of vitamin D are common across all age groups in the UK. In theory, eating two portions of oily fish a week and getting out in the sun for 15 minutes (without sunscreen) each day when it shines will mean you get enough, but not many people do this. Toddlers, pregnant and breast-feeding women and the elderly are groups the Department of Health specifically recommends should take a 10-microgram supplement. In America, the Institute of Medicine recommends that all adults should consume 15 micrograms of vitamin D a day, and that over 70s should have 20 micrograms from food and/or supplements.

People who rarely get out in the sun, have dark skin, or keep their skin covered at all times are particularly likely to need supplements of vitamin D, especially if their intake of oily fish is low. Very low levels of vitamin D may manifest as generalised aches and pains and over the longer term can contribute to weakened bones. Rickets is a vitamin D deficiency disease of childhood that has been making a reappearance in the UK.

Supplement tips
- Look for vitamin D3 (cholecalciferol) in supplements, rather than vitamin D2 (ergocalciferol), as it's likely to be better absorbed.
- For bone benefits, look for vitamin D teamed with calcium and magnesium.

VITAMIN E

RDA: 12mg; *Safe Upper Level*: 540mg

Vitamin E is sometimes also measured in international units (iu), with 1mg of vitamin E equalling around 1.5iu

Food sources
Sunflower oil and seeds, nuts (particularly hazelnuts and almonds), avocados, tomatoes and blackberries.

What it does
Like other antioxidants, vitamin E helps protect cells against the effects of free radicals and oxidative damage (see 'The Lowdown on Antioxidants', page 57). It may also play a role in immune function. It works synergistically with vitamin C: in

simple terms, vitamin C helps protect the watery inside of the cell, whereas vitamin E helps protect the fatty cell membrane. It used to be thought that high doses of vitamin E (up to 270mg or 400iu) were a protection against heart disease and cancer, but this has subsequently been shown not to be so. However, it's thought (but not proven) that this sort of dose may still be useful (together with other antioxidants) to protect the deterioration of the eyes in people who have macular degeneration. And in an analysis from Harvard University's Women's Health Study, women taking vitamin E every other day for a decade had a 10% reduced risk of chronic lung disease, though two previous clinical trials found no such effect.

Who might need a top-up?

It can be reasonably hard to get the RDA of 12mg from foods, and anyone can fall short if they don't regularly include vegetable oils, nuts and seeds in their diet.

Supplement tips

- Vitamin E is one of the more important vitamins to look for in a multivitamin supplement, so check that it contains 12mg (100% of the RDA).
- There isn't much evidence that taking more is useful, but if you do, there seems little point in taking more than 270mg (400iu) a day (see 'Caution!' below).
- Vitamin E is the only vitamin that is more potent in natural rather than synthesised form. Natural source is denoted by the prefix 'd-' in the ingredients (as in d-alpha tocopherol), whereas synthetic is denoted by the prefix 'dl' (dl-alpha tocopherol). If your product contains natural vitamin E it is going to be around one and a half times more potent than if it contains the dl- form.

Caution!

The Safe Upper Level for vitamin E was set at 540mg (800iu) around ten years ago, but this may no longer be valid. Newer trials have yielded negative or inconclusive results regarding the vitamin, and some evidence suggests that high dose vitamin E supplements might actually be harmful in some circumstances, for example they may be linked with higher prostate cancer risk in men. Most experts would advise you not to take more than 270mg (400iu). Sticking close to the RDA of 12mg is, in fact, probably the best bet for most people.

TOCOPHEROLS AND TOCOTRIENOLS – EIGHT TYPES OF VITAMIN E!

Vitamin E is not one substance, but eight related compounds – four tocopherols (alpha, beta, gamma and delta) plus four tocotrienols (also alpha, beta, gamma, delta). Some supplement manufacturers sell mixed tocopherol supplements, claiming these to be better for the body, but there is little research to back this. Evidence shows that the body will 'sort through' all forms of vitamin E in the liver and preferentially secrete alpha tocopherol into the circulation. If your supplement contains a mixture of tocopherols and tocotrienols with weaker potencies than alpha tocopherol, the 'αTE' equivalent must be worked out and stated on the label, to make sure dosages can be compared across products.

THE LOWDOWN ON ANTIOXIDANTS

It's hard to imagine that not so many years ago, nobody had ever heard the word 'antioxidant'. Now, antioxidants are added to everything from food to face cream, with phrases like 'anti-ageing', 'wrinkle-fighting' and 'immune-boosting' attached. But what are antioxidants, and could the tide be turning against them?

An antioxidant is a substance that can prevent the chemical process of oxidation that damages cells. It's analogous to a kamikaze pilot, sacrificing itself to obliterate free radicals.

Free radicals are highly reactive molecules that steal electrons from other molecules in a bid to become chemically stable. This 'stealing' of electrons, and the biological oxidation that results, causes a cascade of damage in our bodies, such as altering the structure of LDL ('bad') cholesterol so it is more likely to damage arteries, and damaging the genetic material in our cells in a way that may lead to tumours.

Vitamin C, beta carotene (and other carotenoids), vitamin E, selenium and flavonoids (including quercetin) are all part of our antioxidant armour. Because they protect against oxidation, it was hoped that by taking higher dose anti-oxidant supplements we would be able to live longer and slash the rates of diseases like heart disease and cancer. However, despite the plausible mechanism, an extensive review by the respected Cochrane Library (published in 2008) concluded that antioxidant pills do not help, and may even have potential downsides.

The Cochrane study pulled in the results of 67 trials and data on more than 232,000 people, and was the biggest ever meta-review to look at the effect of antioxidant supplementation on mortality. The study found no reduction in mortality rates in people who took antioxidant supplements, either in healthy people or in those with diseases.

Researchers now believe that the antioxidant story is more complex than just 'more is better'. And whilst eating plenty of antioxidant vitamins as part of a healthy fruit- and vegetable-rich diet is disease-protective, high doses of single antioxidants, out of sync with the others, may not be good. One theory is that at high doses, some antioxidants turn from antioxidant (quenching free radicals) to pro-oxidant (actually promoting free radicals). Another theory is that constantly damping down free radicals with high doses of antioxidants isn't good, as some free radicals are actually essential for health – for the functioning of the immune system, for example.

So are there any situations where higher dose antioxidant supplements are still good? One area might be for macular degeneration, and another for fertility; a review showed that women were more likely to have a pregnancy or live birth if their partner took antioxidants. There's every reason to supplement with modest amounts of antioxidant nutrients if you are deficient in them. But for general health and future well-being, less may be more, and taking doses of antioxidants that are many times more than the RDA for the long term may not be wise.

VITAMIN K

RDA: 75µg; *Safe Upper Level*: 1000µg

Food sources
Green vegetables, especially leafy salad types. This vitamin can also be made by your intestinal bacteria, so it is not deemed absolutely necessary to have a dietary source.

What it does
Vitamin K plays a crucial role in helping blood to clot. Without vitamin K, the smallest cut could be devastating and result in haemorrhage. There's growing evidence that vitamin K is important for healthy, strong bones too.

Who might need a top-up?
It is very rare under normal circumstances that adults fall short of vitamin K. But you might have low levels if you eat very low amounts of green veg.

Supplement tips
A good multivitamin will contain from 20 micrograms up to the RDA (75µg) of vitamin K.

Caution!
If you're on blood-thinning drugs such as warfarin, you should check with your doctor before taking a supplement that contains vitamin K.

MINERALS

CALCIUM

RDA: 800mg; *Safe Upper Level*: 1500mg

Food sources
Dairy foods like milk, cheese and yoghurt are amongst the best sources of calcium, but it's also found in nuts such as almonds, canned fish with bones, and leafy greens such as watercress and spring greens. Non-dairy alternatives, including soya and rice milk, are also commonly fortified with the mineral.

What it does
A mineral vital for bone health, calcium is also needed for many other bodily functions, such as regulating the heart-beat, conducting nerve impulses, and making muscles contract. Almost all the calcium in the body is found in bone and teeth. Some studies have linked high calcium intakes to lower body weight or less weight gain over time, as well as lower blood pressure.

Who might need a top-up?
The UK's National Diet and Nutrition Survey suggests at least one in five girls and one in eight women have inadequate calcium intakes, probably through not eating the recommended two to three daily portions of dairy products (men and boys are less likely to be deficient). If you suffer with menstrual woes you may particularly want to look at righting a low calcium intake, as low levels of the mineral may contribute to PMS.

Breast-feeding women may need calcium supplements, as this group is recommended to have 1250mg of calcium per day, which can be hard to get from food alone. The National

Osteoporosis Society suggests that people taking osteoporosis drug treatments might also benefit from increasing their daily calcium intake to a total of 1000mg, whilst America's Institute of Medicine recommends women over 50 consume 1200mg per day.

Supplement tips

- Make sure your calcium supplement also contains some vitamin D to help with calcium absorption (or at least check you're getting the vitamin D from somewhere else, if not in the calcium product itself).
- Split any dose that's above 500mg into two or three doses throughout the day.
- If you're taking your calcium with meals, calcium carbonate is fine. If you're not always able to do this, or you have digestive difficulties, look for calcium citrate, which doesn't require stomach acid to break it down.

Caution!

Though the Safe Upper Level for calcium is 1500mg, more recent evidence flags some potential issues with taking too much of this mineral every day. For example, a study in the *British Medical Journal* found that women taking calcium supplements on top of a high dietary calcium intake (1400mg plus a day) were at increased risk of dying from heart disease. A high intake of calcium from supplements, but not foods, may also be associated with an increased risk of kidney stones. For this reason, it's probably best not to exceed a supplemental dose of 1000mg–1200mg of calcium. On days when you eat lots of calcium-rich foods, you can reduce or skip the supplement.

BORON AND SILICON – BONE HELPERS?

Boron and silicon don't have an RDA, and it's still not known if either mineral is truly essential for human health. However, both are allowed in supplements, where they are often teamed with calcium and vitamin D in 'osteo'-style products marketed for bones and joints. Certainly they would seem to be potentially helpful for a healthy skeleton, with boron (found in foods like leafy vegetables, raisins, prunes, nuts and grains) helping assist in the proper absorption of calcium and magnesium and slowing the loss of these minerals in the urine. Silicon, meanwhile, helps the body produce collagen and glycosaminoglycans, essential for healthy bone, nails, hair and skin. Up to 6mg (some authorities say 10mg) of boron per day is deemed safe, and a supplement that contains in the region of 10mg–30mg of silicon a day is also most likely safe, as this amount is similar to the 10mg–40mg a day consumed in a typical diet.

CHROMIUM

RDA: 40µg; *Safe Upper Level*: 10mg

Food sources

Chromium is widely distributed in the food supply, but most foods provide only small amounts per serving. Meat and wholegrain foods, as well as some fruits and vegetables (broccoli, red and black grapes and red wine), are relatively good sources.

What it does

Chromium is thought to enhance the action of insulin, a hormone that is critical to the metabolism and storage of carbohydrate, fat and protein in the body. More research is needed to determine the full range of its roles in the body. It's been suggested, but not proven, that taking chromium supplements may be useful in cutting food cravings.

Who might need a top-up?

People who eat highly refined or very sugary diets are thought to be more at risk from marginal chromium intakes. Older people are also thought more vulnerable to chromium depletion, but chromium status is difficult to determine so it's not possible to be sure. Lower levels in diabetics may make blood sugar control more difficult, so if you have diabetes it's important you make sure that you get enough.

Supplement tips

- Making sure your multivitamin contains up to 40 micrograms of chromium (100% of the RDA) would seen sensible, so you know you are getting enough.
- Nobody knows if higher levels offer bigger benefits but if you want to give it a go, stay within the Safe Upper Level (10mg).
- Chromium in the form of chromium picolinate was once thought to be a cancer risk, but the Food Standards Agency revised its opinion, on advice from the Committee on Mutagenicity, and now says this form of the mineral is safe.

COPPER

RDA: 1mg; *Safe Upper Level*: 10mg

Food sources

Many foods contain some copper. Nuts, shellfish and liver are amongst the richest sources.

What it does

Copper has many functions, but is particularly involved in producing red blood cells that carry oxygen around the body. It is thought to be important for infant growth, brain development, the immune system and strong bones.

Who might need a top-up?

Most people should get enough through their diet, and there's little concern about copper deficiency in the British diet.

Supplement tips

Look for up to 1mg copper (100% of the RDA) in a multivitamin supplement as a nutritional safeguard.

IRON

RDA: 14mg; *Safe Upper Level*: 17mg

Food sources

Liver, meat, beans, dried fruit, nuts (e.g. cashews) and green leafy veg. Spinach is often thought of as a good source of iron, but it also contains oxalic acid, which interferes with iron absorption, so it's not brilliant as an iron source. Tea and coffee can also interfere with iron absorption, which means that people with a vulnerable iron status (such as women who have heavy periods) should avoid drinking them with meals.

What it does

Iron is an essential mineral that becomes incorporated into the haemoglobin of red blood cells, which carry oxygen around the body. A lack of iron can lead to anaemia, with symptoms that include weariness and fatigue, poor concentration, pale skin and hair loss.

Who might need a top-up?

Up to 30% of teenage girls and 17% of women are affected by a low iron status. In the government's National Diet and Nutrition Survey, 46% of girls aged between 11 and 18 and 23% of women aged between 19 and 64 had inadequate intakes of the mineral, probably though low intakes of lean red meats, which provide the best-absorbed form of iron.

Supplement tips

- A multivitamin taken by premenopausal women should include 14mg of iron (100% of the RDA).
- If you're actually diagnosed with anaemia, take the iron that you will be prescribed – doctors can give higher levels of iron than are available over the counter.
- Men might want to consider a supplement without iron, or at least to watch that they don't get more than the RDA across the supplements they take. If you don't need the extra iron, too much can prove harmful because the free iron can accumulate in organs and tissues and may act as a catalyst to damaging oxidation reactions in the body.

IODINE

RDA: 150µg; *Safe Upper Level*: 500µg

Food sources

Fish and dairy products are by far the two biggest sources of iodine.

What it does

Iodine is vital for the formation of thyroid hormones that control metabolic rate. It's also vital to a baby's brain development in the womb and low levels have the potential to affect

IQ. Worryingly, experts at the University of Surrey and the University of Bristol recently found that two-thirds of the pregnant women in the study were iodine deficient.

Who might need a top-up?

Women and girls in particular need to consider how much they are getting; 10% of women between 19 and 64 and 20% of girls aged between 11 and 18 have levels of intake that put them at high risk of deficiency. Making sure you have a couple of dairy portions a day and eating fish a couple of times a week is enough to address a low intake. However, the NHS Choices website has recently added guidance that pregnant women may need to take iodine supplements.

Supplement tips

Don't overlook this mineral – a good multi should always provide 150 micrograms of iodine.

MAGNESIUM

RDA: 375mg; *Safe Upper Level*: 400mg

Food sources

Wholegrain and high-fibre foods, such as wholemeal bread and bran cereals (especially All Bran), nuts (especially Brazils), beans, seeds, fish, avocados, bananas and leafy greens such as spinach.

What it does

Magnesium is an important component of bones (helping to keep them strong), is involved in energy production, helps with muscle contraction and helps keep heart and blood vessels healthy. A magnesium deficiency can impair the body's use of calcium and vitamin D.

Who might need a top-up?

Virtually anyone is vulnerable to a magnesium deficiency as although there is plenty of food with low to medium levels of the mineral, there are few really rich food sources. Eleven per cent of women (aged between 19 and 50), 16% of men and a whopping 28% and 51% respectively of teenage boys and girls can be considered at high risk of magnesium deficiency, according to National Diet and Nutrition Survey data. Older people tend to absorb less of the mineral, so are also at risk. Low magnesium levels have been implicated in migraines, restless leg syndrome, premenstrual syndrome and poor sugar control in people with diabetes, so if you suffer with any of these it's worth considering if you're getting enough from your diet, and, if not, to take a supplement.

Supplement tips

- An A–Z multivitamin and mineral can do a good basic job of topping up marginally deficient intakes, as long as it contains a minimum of around 50mg of magnesium.
- You'll need higher levels if you are looking to tackle a specific health issue.
- If you're taking magnesium for bones, make sure it's teamed with other important bone nutrients such as calcium and vitamin D.

MANGANESE

RDA: 2mg; *Safe Upper Level*: 4mg

Food sources

Whole grains, avocados, pulses, dark chocolate, egg yolks, nuts, seeds, pineapples and green vegetables. Maple syrup is also a tasty source of manganese.

What it does
Manganese plays a particularly important role as part of the natural antioxidant enzyme superoxide dismutase (SOD), which helps fight the damaging free radicals. It also helps energy metabolism, thyroid function, blood sugar control and the formation of collagen, a connective tissue that helps to hold your body together and supports bone and joint health.

Who might need a top-up?
If you need to take high doses of iron or calcium, it would be a good idea to top up your manganese as well (the mineral can be depleted by high levels of these two).

Supplement tips
Manganese is generally only available in supplement form in multivitamins – look for 25% of the RDA or above.

MOLYBDENUM

RDA: 50µg; *Safe Upper Level*: 200µg

Food sources
Dairy products, whole grains, peas, beans and tofu.

What it does
Molybdenum assists in the function of a number of enzymes (proteins that help chemical reactions to take place) in the body. It is considered important for normal cell function and growth, but claims that the mineral can help with libido and tooth decay are unfounded.

Who might need a top-up?
There's no reason to think that most people's intake of this

mineral isn't adequate. And there are no known uses of molybdenum that would suggest doses other than around the RDA.

Supplement tips
The most complete multivitamins will contain up to 100% of the RDA of molybdenum.

POTASSIUM
RDA: 2000mg; *Safe Upper Level*: 3700mg

Food sources
All fruits and vegetables, especially potatoes, bananas, orange juice and avocados, supply potassium, and the mineral is also in nuts, dairy products, meat and fish.

What it does
Potassium levels in the body are tightly controlled, as a correct potassium/sodium balance is needed to keep the right amount of fluid both in and outside cells. An adequate potassium level combined with a modest salt (sodium) intake can help to keep blood pressure healthy.

Who might need a top-up?
You could be a bit low in potassium if you don't get your 5-a-day fruit and veg. Average intake in the UK is above the RDA of 2000mg, though nearly a quarter of women and around 10% of men consume less than this.

Supplement tips
- It's generally agreed that getting potassium from food is the most efficient and safest way to get the mineral.
- If you do find it in a supplement there will be nowhere

near the RDA as you simply can't fit that much in a pill. It's better to top up with some fruit and veg instead.

SELENIUM

RDA: 55µg; *Safe Upper Level*: 350µg

Food sources
Brazil nuts are by far the best source of selenium. You'll find plenty in tinned tuna too.

What it does
Selenium is required for a well-functioning immune system, and one study found that in healthy people in Britain (where marginally low selenium intake is common), selenium supplements improved general immune function, as measured by response to poliovirus immunisation. It's been surmised that selenium helps protect against the development of cancer and perhaps rheumatoid arthritis. If this is the case it only appears to apply to people who are selenium deficient; adding more selenium to a selenium-replete diet makes no difference. Interestingly, a 2008 study at America's Mayo Clinic looked at the effect of selenium supplementation on cancer risk and found that there was a benefit in men, but not women.

Who might need a top-up?
A lot of people are likely to be a bit short in this mineral, given that the average daily intake of selenium in the UK (from National Diet and Nutrition Survey data) is 42 micrograms in women and 53 micrograms in men.

Supplement tips
Check your multivitamin contains some – 100% of the RDA

is ideal. But even a smaller amount – such as 20–50% of the RDA – will still provide a valuable top-up.

Caution!

Selenium is one of those minerals where there's not too much difference between a safe dose and a harmful one. The safe upper limit is 350 micrograms, and more than a 900 microgram dose can cause nausea and vomiting, and maybe hair and nail loss and depression in the long term. Preliminary research indicates that taking 200 micrograms daily on top of a high-selenium diet may raise the risk of diabetes.

ZINC

RDA: 10mg; *Safe Upper Level*: 25mg

Food sources

Red meats such as lamb and beef, crab, sardines, nuts (especially pecans) and whole grains such as wholemeal bread and whole wheat pasta.

What it does

Zinc is an essential mineral found in almost every cell and is needed for cell division, growth, wound healing, and proper functioning of the immune system. The mineral also plays a role in taste and smell. It isn't in itself an antioxidant, but it supports antioxidant processes in the body. A 2012 review from the Cochrane Library showed that sucking zinc lozenges can shorten colds by about a day and reduce the severity of symptoms, particularly when started within 24 hours of the cold's onset. The same review found that zinc supplementation for at least five months reduced incidence of the common cold in children and the number of school absences taken.

A decade ago a well-designed study found that a supplement containing zinc and antioxidants (see also 'Lutein', page 95) could help people diagnosed with age-related macular degeneration (AMD). The original zinc dose was a hefty 80mg (more than the Safe Upper Level), but results from a recent update of the study (known as AREDS2 – Age-Related Eye Disease Study 2) used 25mg, which was a useful dose too.

Who might need a top-up?

Teenagers can often have low intakes of zinc, and you need more of the vitamin when you are breast-feeding. If you're constantly getting colds or infections, have jaded taste buds or wounds that are slow to heal, it could be a sign that your intake is a bit low. If you are a strict vegetarian, or over 60, you may also need to top up your intake.

Supplement tips

- Look for 10mg a day in multi formulations – there's rarely a good reason for you to need more than this.
- If you want to try zinc lozenges when you have a cold, start as soon as you have symptoms and follow the dosing advice on the label (usually one lozenge every two to four hours). This is a bit of a shot in the dark, as there's too little research to pin down exactly the dose or formulation that works best. However, there's some indication that zinc acetate or zinc gluconate are best, so you could look for these on the label.

NOT SO MAGIC MINERALS

PHOSPHORUS

Though this mineral is essential and will often appear in multivitamin and mineral formulations, most people get plenty of phosphorus in their diets. If you're getting a disproportionately high amount of phosphorus compared to calcium, it could lead to bone loss. The safe maximum amount in a supplement is 250mg (less than the RDA).

SODIUM

Sodium is allowed in supplements, but you really don't want any extra sodium as it is the chemical constituent of salt (sodium chloride), which raises blood pressure.

FLUORIDE

This mineral is important for bones and teeth but has always been controversial, with very polarised views over whether adding it to water (as is done in some areas of the UK) is 'mass medication' or not. Fluoride is allowed in supplements but most manufacturers stay clear of it, and tea drinkers already get plenty. For active protection against tooth decay, fluoride also needs to actually come into direct contact with the teeth, so supplements are less relevant.

5
POPULAR HERBS

ST JOHN'S WORT

A tall plant with yellow flowers, St John's wort (*Hypericum perforatum*) has been used as a tonic for 'nerves' for hundreds of years.

Who might need St John's wort?

People with mild to moderate depression who do not want to take, or cannot tolerate, prescription antidepressants are the group who are most likely to benefit from a supplement of St John's wort.

What are the benefits?

St John's wort is one of the most well-researched herbal medicines. Results aren't entirely consistent, but studies show that if it's taken in the right form and in the correct dosage it can act as an effective treatment for people with mild to moderate depression. Its mode of action is thought very similar to the modern SSRI (selective serotonin re-uptake inhibitor) drugs such as Prozac, and its effect in the brain is to lift levels of important mood-enhancing brain chemicals, such as serotonin, dopamine and noradrenalin.

Tips on choosing and using

- St John's wort is available as a registered traditional herbal medicine, so look for this certification (the letters THR and a leaf symbol in a black square) on the label. It's a simple first-line strategy to guarantee the safety and purity of herbal products.
- Effective products will contain a concentrated extract of St John's wort with a standardised amount (0.3% usually) of the active ingredient, hypericin. Look for doses of between 300mg and 900mg of St John's wort extract to deliver the right amount of this active ingredient.

Safety

St John's wort has to be used with the same caution as prescription SSRI antidepressants and can interfere with a variety of drugs, including statins, blood thinners and oral contraceptives, amongst others. Side effects include nausea upon first taking the herb, allergic skin reactions and hypersensitivity to sunlight. If you're on any medication it's always best to check with your doctor before taking St John's wort. Needless to say, it must not be taken with drugs that have been prescribed for depression.

GINSENG

Another quite well-researched herb, Asian or Chinese ginseng, also known as Panax ginseng, was traditionally used in Chinese medicine to strengthen the digestion and the lungs, calm the spirit, and increase overall energy. There's a hint of its traditional 'cure all' reputation in the name 'Panax', which means 'all healing' in Greek. The active ingredients are thought to be compounds called ginsenosides.

Who might need ginseng?

Traditionally people under physical and mental stress have taken ginseng, and there is some evidence that you could benefit if your immune system needs a boost. Diabetics might find that they benefit too, though if you have diabetes you should always talk to your doctor before trying anything that could potentially affect your blood sugar.

What are the benefits?

Benefits are hard to evaluate, given there are so many potencies of products available and because ginseng is now largely used in a concentrated extract form, whereas in the old days, when it gained its super-healthy reputation, ginseng tended to be used in its whole root form and in combination with other herbs. That said, there's 'B grade' (good) evidence, according to the Natural Standard – an international research collaboration that systematically reviews scientific evidence on complementary and alternative medicine – that ginseng can boost the immune system. There's similarly quite good evidence that ginseng might help control blood sugar, though not every study has shown this. And there are some reasonably good-quality studies showing that ginseng may help mental function, as well as possible erectile function in males.

Tips on choosing and using

- It's particularly important that you buy ginseng from a reputable source, as Chinese herbal remedies have been those that have been most troubled by contamination and safety issues. Check products are standardised on their ginsenoside content, or look for products with a 'THR' (traditional herbal medicine registration) kitemark.
- A typical dosage is about 500mg to 2000mg of ginseng root equivalent daily. (The term 'equivalent' is needed

because the ginseng in supplements is usually a concentrated extract. For example, it may be a 10:1 concentration, such that 100mg in the tablet is equivalent to 1000mg of actual ginseng root.) You might need at least 2000mg root equivalent daily to boost mental function.

Safety
Ginseng may react with blood-thinning medication, insulin and some antidepressants, and should be used with caution by those with high blood pressure. Long-term use may be connected with anxiety and insomnia.

GINKGO BILOBA

Ginkgo biloba (or just ginkgo for short), is an ancient Chinese remedy that comes from the leaves of the *Ginkgo biloba* (maidenhair) tree. Popular in Germany, where it is a prescribed medicine, its active ingredient, ginkgo flavone glycosides, has been shown to improve circulation.

Who might need ginkgo?
If you have poor circulation or cognitive impairment you might benefit from a supplement of this herb.

What are the benefits?
Ginkgo is a bit like aspirin, in that it may help stop blood clots from forming and may increase blood flow. The standardised form of ginkgo, which was developed in Germany and has been used in many clinical trials, is prescribed for 'cerebral insufficiency', which can cover everything from confusion, anxiety and depression to headaches and intermittent claudication (pain in the legs due to insufficient blood flow).

DOES BETTER BLOOD FLOW
MEAN A PERKIER BRAIN?

It was once thought that ginkgo probably helped mental function by improving circulation of blood to the brain. But though improvement in circulation may certainly play a role, the up-to-date understanding of age-related memory loss no longer considers blood flow a primary issue. Most things that help dementia may instead function by directly stimulating nerve cell activity and by protecting nerve cells from further injury.

In truth the evidence is limited for most of these, and most of the research into ginkgo has been carried out in the area of Alzheimer's and dementia. Scientific evidence is equivocal here too, though. For example, a small Italian study in 2006 found ginkgo as effective as a conventional drug treatment (Aricept) in cases of mild to moderate Alzheimer's. A German study in 2012 also found that ginkgo improved brain function and behavioural problems better than a placebo in mild to moderate Alzheimer's. But other studies have given negative results.

Combining ginkgo with Panax ginseng could be a good move if you're feeling forgetful. There's some evidence that the two together can improve memory in otherwise healthy people between the ages of 38 and 66, according to the Natural Medicines' Comprehensive Database – another respected source rating the effectiveness of herbal and other remedies.

Tips on choosing and using
- The effective daily dosage, proven by clinical trials, is 100mg–150mg of a ginkgo extract which provides 24% of the main active ingredient, ginkgo flavone glycosides.

- If you can't find this information on the label, look for a 'THR' logo, which means it is a registered traditional herbal medicine and has been formulated to high standards.

Safety
Rare side effects include headache, palpitations and dizziness. Take care if you're on blood-thinning drugs.

OTHER HERBS FOR YOUR MENTAL WELL-BEING

Ginkgo and ginseng are the herbs most often thought of in relation to mental function, but a new kid on the block is *rhodiola*, which preliminary evidence seems to suggest might help deal with anxiety and stress-induced fatigue. *Passionflower* (also known as *passiflora*) is another potential anxiety-reliever, and for a gentle sleep aid it's worth trying *valerian*. All should be taken according to the label information and any possible contraindications of side effects noted.

ECHINACEA

Traditionally used as a treatment for colds, echinacea, also known as purple coneflower, can contain the leaves and roots of various *Echinacea* species, part of the daisy family.

Who might need echinacea?
If you're coming down with a cold, or trying to fight one off, echinacea could be a herbal product for you to try.

What are the benefits?

According to a 2009 review by the respected Cochrane Library, 'there is some evidence that preparations based on the aerial parts of *Echinacea purpurea* might be effective for the early treatment of colds in adults but the results are not fully consistent.'

More impressively, a Swiss liquid echinacea extract, which included both the leaves and flowers, reduced the number and severity of colds by a very respectable 25%, compared with a placebo, in a Cardiff University study in 2012. But the results have been criticised because of deficiencies in the report writing and because the study was part-funded by the manufacturer but not declared. Other individual studies and reviews suggest either minor positive effects or no effect at all. But the exact formulation and dosage of the herb seem to be of key importance.

As with all drugs and supplements, believing echinacea will help you means it probably will. In one 2011 study at the University of Wisconsin, people with colds benefited most if they believed echinacea was effective, and this applied whether they were given the active treatment or a placebo.

Tips on choosing and using

- Use a product that contains *Echinacea purpurea*, as this is the most studied form (though *Echinacea angustifolia* may also be OK).
- The dosage of extract that you should look for should be equivalent to about 2000mg–4000mg of the fresh echinacea herb.
- An echinacea product that's classified as a registered traditional herbal medicine is best.
- Don't take it all the time – the recommended maximum period is ten days, though courses can be repeated over the cold season if necessary, with short breaks in between.

Safety

Studies have not shown any significant toxicity of echinacea. However, people who are allergic to daisies, marigolds and other plants in the *Asteraceae* family should not use it. The potential that an allergic reaction could be very serious is greater in children and for this reason the UK Medicines and Healthcare Products Regulatory Agency (MHRA) recently advised that echinacea should not be given to children under 12.

IS PELARGONIUM THE NEW ECHINACEA?

Also being hailed for its potential to see off respiratory troubles is the herb pelargonium. The herb has already shown promise in reducing asthma, acute bronchitis, coughs and colds, but more recently it has given hope to sufferers of the more debilitating condition, chronic obstructive pulmonary disease (COPD). More work needs to be done, but in a high-quality study, COPD sufferers who took the herb had a longer time between flare-ups, took fewer antibiotics and had a better quality of life compared with those given a placebo.

BLACK COHOSH

A herbal product that has become more popular in recent years, black cohosh has its roots in Native American history, being long used to treat 'women's complaints'.

Who might need black cohosh?

This herb appeals particularly to women because of its historical use in balancing hormones.

What are the benefits?

Over 50 components in black cohosh have potential biological effects that could include oestrogen-like effects, analgesic properties and an influence on serotonin levels in the brain. Some but not all studies have suggested that black cohosh can help deal with hot flushes and, based on its traditional use, well-formulated black cohosh products can be licensed as traditional herbal medicines for menopausal symptoms. Bear in mind, however, that this certification only gives a guarantee of quality and not necessarily of efficacy.

Tips on choosing and using

- Choose a product that is a registered traditional herbal medicine, as there have been issues with the quality of black cohosh in the past, with some products containing contaminants.

AGNUS CASTUS FOR TROUBLESOME PERIODS

Younger women experiencing symptoms of PMS (such as breast discomfort, irritability and depression) will find a herb called agnus castus (also known as chasteberry and vitex) a more appropriate option than black cohosh. There is reasonably good evidence that it can soothe PMS, and is also worth trying if you have irregular periods. Agnus castus is thought to work by suppressing the release of prolactin from the pituitary gland. Prolactin is a hormone that naturally rises during pregnancy to stimulate milk production, but inappropriately increased production may be a factor in cyclic breast tenderness, and some forms of irregular menstruation.

- A daily dosage that's equivalent to at least 40mg of black cohosh root is the amount recommended.

Safety

There isn't clear data on the safety of black cohosh, but on the plus side it is not likely to be a herb that a woman would take for years on end. Use of contraception is recommended when you use black cohosh (even if your periods have stopped), as there is the outside chance that its hormonal effects could increase your fertility.

SOME OTHER POPULAR HERBS

MILK THISTLE

Evidence from studies in animals suggests that milk thistle can protect the liver from numerous toxins. Reasons you might want to try it include if you've been drinking too much alcohol or as an extra protection when taking medications known to cause liver problems.

ARTICHOKE LEAF

Artichoke leaf is a popular folk hangover cure, but a small, double-blind, placebo-controlled study published in the *Canadian Medical Association Journal* failed to find artichoke more effective than a placebo at beating morning-after symptoms. However, at least one substantial study indicates that artichoke leaf is helpful for dealing with 'dyspepsia' – a term that includes discomfort in the stomach, bloating, lack of appetite, nausea and mild diarrhoea or constipation.

SAW PALMETTO

Some evidence suggests that saw palmetto might be useful for men with an enlarged prostate (also known as benign prostatic hypertrophy or BPH). It may help with urgent or frequent urination, but men should always discuss any urinary symptoms with their doctor, as they need to have a proper diagnosis of their condition.

DEVIL'S CLAW

South Africans have traditionally used devil's claw to reduce pain and fever and in European countries it has became a popular treatment for arthritis. According to the Natural Medicines' Comprehensive Database, devil's claw is 'possibly effective' for decreasing pain from osteoarthritis. There is insufficient evidence in the use of devil's claw in rheumatoid arthritis.

FEVERFEW

This herb is a traditional remedy for migraine, but if it is effective at all (and some evidence shows it does reduce production of hormone-like substances called prostaglandins that play a role in producing pain sensations), you need to take it every day. Regular use for several months may help as a preventative, but it won't help as a pain reliever if your head already aches.

6
OTHER POPULAR SUPPLEMENTS

PROBIOTICS

The term 'probiotic' refers to dietary supplements (tablets, capsules, powders and dairy drinks) that contain 'friendly' gut bacteria. The two commonest types that are used are *Lactobacilli* and *Bifidobacteria*, but there are many different sub-strains, with potentially different effects. Overall, though, the idea of taking probiotic supplements is that you outweigh 'bad' bacteria with 'good' types, keeping the digestive system healthy. Research has revealed that having a healthy balance of gut bacteria is also vital to a healthy immune system.

Who might need probiotics?
If you've been on a course of antibiotics you could benefit from probiotics to repopulate your gut with healthy bacteria and help prevent rebound infections (such as thrush and stomach bugs). There's some evidence that if you have irritable bowel syndrome you might be helped by a probiotic too, and if you're travelling abroad where you can't guarantee the food hygiene standards there's also logic to taking one. Older people tend to have natural reductions in healthy gut bacteria, so they also are likely to benefit.

What are the benefits?

It's fair to say that there are an awful lot of unknowns, as there are so many different probiotic strains and different people will respond in different ways to different products, depending on the bowel bacteria they have to begin with, their immune status and other factors. However, there is good evidence that probiotics can help ease infectious diarrhoea and diarrhoea caused by antibiotic use. Two reviews from 2012, one in the *Journal of the American Medical Association* and one in the *Annals of Internal Medicine* – which together included more than 80 studies and 14,000 people – found that probiotic therapy reduced the risk of antibiotic-associated diarrhoea (including that caused by the bacterium *Clostridium difficile*, which can be life-threatening) by 42% and 66%, respectively.

Some studies suggest that specific probiotic strains can also help in mild to moderate ulcerative colitis (a type of inflammatory bowel disease) and irritable bowel syndrome. Some strains have been shown to improve stool consistency, for example, or increase frequency of bowel movements in those where constipation was a major symptom.

In the area of immune health, probiotics have been linked to enhanced immune responses to vaccines (such as to flu vaccines). A 2011 review by the respected Cochrane Library concluded that probiotics might also be beneficial for preventing acute respiratory infections, though there were limitations in the studies and no data for older people. One of the actions of probiotics seems to be to help dampen down the immune system so it doesn't overreact to stimuli that are not harmful. Along these lines there are some studies that suggest that taking probiotics in pregnancy may help to reduce the likelihood of a baby developing the autoimmune condition eczema. Other studies conclude that probiotics make no difference, or that there's just not enough evidence either way.

Tips on choosing and using

- Always stick to bacterial strains that start with the names *Lactobacillus* or *Bifidobacterium*. There are other genera of bacteria, including yeasts and cocci, which can be described as 'friendly' but are less proven in their effects.
- A product should have an absolute minimum of 10 million bacteria per dose. If it doesn't state the bacterial count on the label, check with the manufacturer – or don't bother with it.
- If you want a probiotic that will deliver more strongly on gut benefits, choose one containing largely *Bifidobacteria*.
- For immune-enhancing effects (including against colds), one containing *Lactobacilli* or *Lactobacilli* and *Bifidobacteria* combined is suitable.
- The most effective probiotic will also contain a decent dose (at least 2g) of 'prebiotic' (see below).

PREBIOTICS

Pick up a probiotic supplement and you could find it's got 'prebiotic' written somewhere on the label too. This isn't a spelling mistake – prebiotics are separate entities that work alongside probiotics to increase the number of good bugs in your gut. They are indigestible plant fibres, such as galacto-oligosaccharides, fructo-oligosaccharides and inulin, which *Bifidobacteria* use as a food source, multiplying substantially as a result of gobbling them up. In fact, adding prebiotics to probiotics has been described a bit like the good bugs taking their lunch boxes down with them! Prebiotics occur naturally in foods such as leeks, onions, asparagus, bananas, chicory and Jerusalem artichokes, so you can also boost the number of good bugs naturally by eating a diet rich in these vegetables.

Safety

Probiotics may cause mild gut disturbances such as wind or loose bowel movements in some users at first but they shouldn't cause any problems in people who are generally healthy. However, probiotics may be less safe in very ill or immunocompromised individuals and they shouldn't be given in these situations without medical advice.

COENZYME Q10

Coenzyme Q10 (CoQ10) is also called ubiquinone because it belongs to a class of compounds called quinones and is ubiquitous in living creatures. This substance, which can't be classified as a vitamin as the body can make its own supply, plays a crucial role in producing energy in cells and is also a powerful antioxidant.

Who might need CoQ10?

CoQ10 is one of the many substances that tend to decline in the body as the result of ageing or illness. So older people are more likely to be low in it, and people with heart conditions, Parkinson's disease and asthma have also been shown to generally have lower levels. Statins, beta-blockers and antidepressants can also reduce CoQ10 in the body. Lower levels aren't the cause of these diseases, nor is it possible to say that supplementing with CoQ10 will help in tackling them. But there is certainly a lot of research going on into CoQ10 and its potential benefits in areas to do with the heart, muscles and energy release.

What are the benefits?

Some evidence suggests that CoQ10 might assist the heart during times when the heart muscle is under stress, perhaps by helping it use energy more efficiently. In Japan and several European countries it's prescribed (as an adjunct to other medications) for certain heart ailments, and in particular for congestive heart failure.

If you have high blood pressure, taking CoQ10 could also possibly help you, with a review of trials, published in the *Journal of Human Hypertension* in 2007, finding that CoQ10 lowered systolic blood pressure by 11–17 points and diastolic blood pressure by 8–10 points. There is, additionally, some evidence that CoQ10 may reduce the risk of pre-eclampsia (high blood pressure during pregnancy) in women who are at risk for this condition, but pregnant women should talk to their doctor before taking CoQ10.

If you are taking statins for high cholesterol you may be recommended to take a high dose CoQ10 supplement to help minimise the potential side effects of the drug. Some cardiologists believe that it is a drop in CoQ10 levels that brings about the muscle pain and weakness that many statin users complain of and which can very much reduce their quality of life. It's important to take advice from your doctor or consultant, however, as there are many types of statins with different side-effect profiles, meaning that the first route of action may be to change your drug.

Another condition that CoQ10 might potentially help with is Parkinson's disease. Conflicting evidence suggests that high strength supplementation during the early stages may slow progression of the disease, but better-designed studies are needed to confirm this one way or the other. Again, talk to your doctor or consultant, as if you do take CoQ10, large doses may be needed.

Despite very many 'miracle' health claims for CoQ10, if you're already well and healthy there's no reason to think CoQ10 will give you more energy or somehow optimise your health. If you want to optimise the amount you get through diet rather than supplements, make sure you eat lean red meat. Venison is a particularly rich source.

Tips on choosing and using

- Most products on the market contain from 30mg to 200mg CoQ10. It's hard to give specific advice on what levels to take as the information is lacking, but if you're trying to tackle a specific health issue, such as statin side effects, it's likely to be the higher end dosages that are needed.
- Some manufacturers produce what's dubbed a more 'body ready' form of CoQ10 called ubiquinol (rather than ubiquinone). It's argued that this is more easily absorbed and utilised by the body, but it also tends to be more expensive. You could look out for it if you are an older person with digestive troubles.
- Take CoQ10 with a meal as it will be better absorbed this way.

Safety

No serious side effects have been reported, even at very high doses. Talk to your doctor if you are on blood-thinning medications or diabetes drugs, however. CoQ10's long-term safety is still unknown, so don't take high doses without good reason.

GARLIC

An integral part of Mediterranean and Asian cuisines, garlic has been credited with many health benefits, from reducing cholesterol to acting as a natural antibiotic.

Who might need garlic?

If you're concerned about the health of your heart you might consider consuming more garlic.

What are the benefits?

Garlic, or some of the compounds isolated from it, shows anti-cancer, anti-inflammatory, blood-thinning and cholesterol-lowering effects in laboratory and animal studies, but we still know very little about the effects in humans and what the most beneficial form and dosage might be. One 2012 study using an aged garlic extract showed a reduced severity of colds, and one good-quality trial suggested that 200mg of garlic powder, three times a day, lowered blood pressure slightly in people with high readings. And a well-conducted review of 29 studies involving nearly 1800 participants concluded that garlic (mainly garlic powder) produced 'modest reductions' in total cholesterol levels. The big problem, though, is that garlic supplements come in so many forms with differing chemical constituents, and studies haven't been able to ascertain which is best.

Tips on choosing and using

- It's hard to give advice; however, garlic powder products that state on the label that they are standardised on their content of alliin or allicin are probably closest to how you would eat garlic in food.
- Aged garlic extract (active ingredient s-allyl cysteine) is also produced to high-quality standards and is stomach-friendly and odourless.
- High dose garlic oil capsules are the most likely to cause smell on the skin or breath, so look for additional ingredients such as parsley oil, traditionally used to help make your breath less garlicky.

- Don't forget that garlic is also a delicious culinary ingredient and that eating it as part of your everyday meals is likely to benefit health.

Safety

Garlic is largely safe but can occasionally cause stomach upsets in large amounts. Some garlic supplements could interact with blood-thinners such as warfarin, so check with your doctor if you are on these medications.

LYCOPENE

Part of the carotenoid family (of which beta carotene is also a member), lycopene is the antioxidant that gives the red colour to tomatoes. It is found in smaller amounts in watermelon too.

Who might need lycopene?

It's a supplement you might want to look out for if you don't eat many tomato products, especially if you're over 50.

What are the benefits?

Reports linking lycopene with reduced prostate and breast cancer risks have made headlines, but the evidence is far too weak to rely on. More sturdy evidence suggests that lycopene can help in gum disease and other mouth problems, such as precancerous conditions of the mouth. For reasons that are not at all clear, 4mg of lycopene taken daily in pregnancy appears to reduce the risk of pre-eclampsia. Eating lots of tomato paste rich in lycopene has also been shown to give the skin some natural sun protection.

Tips on choosing and using

Look for supplements that supply 4mg–16mg of lycopene in a daily dose – reflecting the amount you could get by eating a moderate to very large quantity of tomato products every day.

Safety

Lycopene supplements appear safe in dosages that could be obtainable through diet.

LUTEIN

Another antioxidant of the carotenoid family, lutein is a yellow pigment that's found concentrated in the macular pigment in the retina of the eye. We get it from vegetables, particularly kale and spinach.

Who might need lutein?

If you've been diagnosed with age-related macular degeneration (AMD), a supplement of lutein could be useful.

What are the benefits?

Lutein appears to protect the cells responsible for vision from light damage. Recent results from the hugely respected AREDS2 study (the second stage of the Age-Related Eye Disease Study), suggest that lutein and zeaxanthin (another antioxidant that occurs in green and yellow veg, such as sweet-corn), with high doses of zinc (25mg), is an effective way to slow the progression of AMD from early stage to more advanced.

Tips on choosing and using

An effective dose is 10mg. Look for supplements that also contain some zeaxanthin – the AREDS2 formula used 2mg of zeaxanthin along with 10mg of lutein.

Safety
Lutein appears to be safer than beta carotene, the more well-known member of the carotenoid family.

ALPHA LIPOIC ACID

Alpha lipoic acid is a crucial component of the mitochondria (energy-producing machines) in cells, and plays an important role in energy production. Only in 1988 – so fairly recently – was it recognised as an important antioxidant, and it has been exciting the attention of some researchers.

Who might need alpha lipoic acid?
The body makes enough alpha lipoic acid for all the important metabolic functions, but some experts argue that those over 50 should take alpha lipoic acid to ensure there is some 'spare' to act as an antioxidant in cells.

What are the benefits?
These are still largely theoretical, but what makes alpha lipoic acid particularly special is its versatility in helping deactivate a wide range of damaging free radicals in many different types of cell and tissue.

One well-known proponent of alpha lipoic acid is Dr Bruce Ames, professor of Biochemistry and Molecular Biology at the University of California, Berkeley, who helped develop a patented (and much copied) supplement containing alpha lipoic acid. Called Juvenon, it boldly claims to 'rejuvenate ageing cells'. It would be lovely if this turns out to be so, but so far there has not been much in the way of human research to support those claims.

Laboratory and animal studies have yielded some promising results, but how they translate into health in humans has not been adequately studied. Most promising is a potential benefit on preventing diabetic neuropathy – in Germany, alpha lipoic acid is routinely used to treat this condition.

Tips on choosing and using

The recommended amount is usually 200mg–400mg. If you want to give it a go, don't take more than that.

Safety

Alpha lipoic acid would appear very safe, but its long-term effects aren't known and it is worth remembering that high doses of antioxidant vitamins that were once hoped to prolong life and fight disease have proved more than disappointing and occasionally even harmful (see 'The Lowdown on Antioxidants', page 57).

OTHER PURPORTED ANTI-AGEING SUPPLEMENTS

ACETYL-L-CARNITINE

Acetyl-L-carnitine can cross the blood–brain barrier and enter the brain, where it acts as another powerful antioxidant. Professor Ames and his California University colleagues found that teaming a daily dose of 1000mg of the substance with 400mg of alpha lipoic acid enabled elderly rats to function like younger ones, and made dogs smarter.

RESVERATROL

A substance that's found naturally in red wine, red and black grapes, peanuts and blueberries, resveratrol is thought to offer some protection against heart disease, mainly because it has antioxidant and anti-inflammatory effects and may keep arteries flexible. There are hints that it can also potentially minimise some of the damaging metabolic changes (like insulin resistance) that happen in obesity. Recently, however, it was found that a prominent researcher in this area, Dipak Das of the University of Connecticut, had fabricated and falsified data in dozens of published papers on resveratrol. The jury is still out as to its benefits.

PINE BARK EXTRACT

Pine bark extract – including the patented Pycnogenol – provides a range of flavonoid and other botanical antioxidants that in laboratory and animal studies can combat inflammation and knock out some cancer cells. In some European countries it's used to help with 'venous insufficiency' (poor blood flow back to the heart, leading to varicose veins and swollen legs). A small study suggested it could help with menopausal hot flushes, and preliminary evidence indicates it might help with diabetic retinopathy – damage to the retina caused by poor blood sugar control.

CONJUGATED LINOLEIC ACID (CLA)

CLA is actually a form of fat, and a trans fat at that, so you'd expect that it should be left well out of a healthy diet. However, it has some special properties that may actually be good for health. CLA occurs naturally in food, for example full-fat dairy products, to a certain extent, but it would be very difficult to get a dose that has measurable effects in the body that way. Supplements are the only practical source.

Who might need CLA?
It's one to consider if you're losing weight and want to hold on to lean tissue.

What are the benefits?
Some studies have suggested that CLA can help when you're losing weight by improving the body's fat to muscle ratio. One meta-analysis (a systematic statistical review of the data) suggested a dose of 3.2g a day can reduce body fat, but another found minimal benefits at most. Some (but not all) animal and laboratory studies suggest that CLA might help prevent cancer.

Tips on choosing and using
The typical dosages of CLA range from 2g to 4g (2000mg–4000mg) daily. As with all supplements taken at this high a dosage, it is important to purchase a reputable brand, as even very small amounts of toxic contaminants that accidentally find their way into the product could quickly add up.

Safety
Individuals with diabetes or who are at risk for diabetes should not use CLA except under medical supervision. This is because of conflicting results as to its effect on insulin sensitivity.

5-HTP

5-HTP (full name 5-hydroxytryptophan) is derived from the amino acid (protein building block) L-tryptophan. In the body 5-HTP is converted into the brain chemical messenger serotonin.

Who might need 5-HTP?

You might consider supplementing with 5-HTP if you're down in the dumps, or suffer with migraines.

What are the benefits?

As 5-HTP makes serotonin, providing the body with an extra amount of the substance may lift serotonin levels, which is the way many antidepressants work. Several small short-term studies have found that 5-HTP may be as effective as standard antidepressant drugs. It is believed 5-HTP may also help relieve migraines, again through enhancing serotonin levels, but more research needs to be done. Other areas where it has shown promise are weight loss, fibromyalgia and anxiety.

Tips on choosing and using

- Studies show that a helpful dose is 100mg three times a day.
- You should work up to this dosage, and never combine 5-HTP with an antidepressant, particularly SSRI drugs like Prozac.

Safety

Side effects appear to be generally limited to short-term, mild digestive distress and possible allergic reactions. However, 5-HTP isn't safe to use with certain Parkinson's medications. It also has the potential to cause serotonin syndrome (confusion, muscle jerks, loss of coordination) if combined with medications that also raise serotonin levels, such as antidepressants and the pain medication tramadol.

TURMERIC

Turmeric is the spice that gives curry its earthy flavour, and has been credited with all manner of health benefits. It's also been used for thousands of years to treat a variety of conditions. The main active ingredient is curcumin.

Who might need turmeric?

It's hard to say as, despite the long history of traditional use, properly controlled studies on the benefits of turmeric are only in their infancy. However, there are tantalising hints that turmeric could be useful if you have inflammatory conditions such as bowel disease or arthritis.

What are the benefits?

In one Japanese study, people whose ulcerative colitis was in remission took either curcumin – the active ingredient of turmeric – or a placebo, along with conventional medical treatment, for six months. Those who took curcumin had a relapse rate much lower than those who took a placebo. Early evidence suggests high dose turmeric may protect against colon cancer in smokers. Turmeric is also surmised to play a role in inhibiting atherosclerosis, a disease of the arteries that restricts blood flow. In studies of mice, a curcumin-rich diet also appeared to have a slimming effect. The German Commission E, which determines which herbs can be safely prescribed in Germany, has approved turmeric for digestive problems because it encourages bile production. It seems that very high levels are necessary to have effects anywhere other than the region of the gut, though, as tumeric is very poorly absorbed into the bloodstream.

Tips on choosing and using

You should check that a turmeric supplement has a standardised curcumin content – 95% curcumin is very good. By comparison, culinary turmeric powders normally contain only 3–5% curcumin.

Safety

Skin rash and stomach ulcers have been reported after long-term use, and allergic reactions are possible, especially if you're already allergic to ginger, or yellow food colourings. You need to be cautious if you're susceptible to kidney stones, and people taking blood-thinning medications, drugs that suppress the immune system, or regular doses of non-steroidal pain relievers (such as ibuprofen) should avoid turmeric because of the risk of harmful drug interactions. Check with your doctor before taking it if you are on anti-cancer drugs.

QUERCETIN

Quercetin is the one of the flavonoid family of compounds found in plants, and perhaps the best studied for its potential health benefits. It's found in some of the largest amounts in onions, and also in black and green tea and red wine.

Who might need quercetin?

It could be worth a try if you have allergies, such as hay fever, for example.

What are the benefits?

In laboratory studies, quercetin prevents immune cells from releasing histamines, chemicals that cause allergic reactions. On that basis, researchers think that quercetin might help reduce symptoms of allergies such as hay fever, including runny nose, watery eyes, hives, and swelling of the face and lips. However, the evidence is still only theoretical for humans. Quercetin might also have modest effects on blood pressure and cholesterol, and it's thought to be one of the substances in a fruit- and veg-rich diet that could help protect against cancer.

Tips on using and choosing
- A typical dosage is 500mg–1000mg daily.
- A special type of quercetin – quercetin chalcone – is claimed to be absorbed better, but there is little reliable evidence to prove this.

Safety
Pregnant and breast-feeding women and people with kidney disease should avoid quercetin. At high doses (greater than 1g per day) there are some reports of damage to the kidneys. It can interact with various drugs, so check with your doctor before taking it if you are on any medication.

7

AN A–Z OF HEALTH CONDITIONS

Good nutrition has a fundamental effect on our health and well-being, as well as on our ability to resist disease. Mostly it's the totality of a healthy diet with its complex and often poorly understood interaction of components that helps to protect us, but sometimes specific vitamins, minerals or supplements can be identified as playing a particularly important role. The next few pages give a guide to those health issues most likely to respond to nutritional help when things go wrong.

ACNE

Chocolate and chips do not specifically exacerbate acne, but a diet that has what is known as a high glycaemic load – i.e., one high in processed snacks, refined sugar and baked goods – may do. A high glycaemic load comes not simply from eating a lot of carbohydrates, but from eating a lot of refined carbohydrates that release their energy fast and raise insulin levels (one theory is that insulin promotes the male hormone testosterone, which contributes to spot outbreaks). To help, eat modest portions of mainly low glycaemic, unrefined carbs such as pulses, whole oats and barley, and wholemeal and grainy breads.

A deficiency of vitamin A could potentially worsen acne by affecting sebaceous gland activity. Eating plenty of carrots, red peppers, mangos and oily fish will ensure a good intake, but a supplement is a good backup. Finally, think zinc: it helps in skin healing and can be lacking in teenagers, the primary group that suffers with acne. Increasing foods rich in zinc (lean meat, grains and seafood) will help, or look for 10mg in a supplement.

AGE-RELATED MACULAR DEGENERATION (AMD)

This is the commonest cause of age-related sight loss, but studies indicate that some protection can come from a healthy diet, and in particular lots of lutein, which is concentrated in the back of the eye and is found in kale and spinach. If you already have AMD, evidence from the second Age-Related Eye Disease Study (AREDS2) suggests that taking 10mg of lutein, 2mg of zeaxanthin and 25mg of zinc daily may slow down progression to a more advanced stage of the disease.

ASTHMA

A Mediterranean diet may be asthma-protective, and it's always good for general health reasons to eat lots of fruits and vegetables, pulses, nuts and oily fish anyway. If you really can't stomach fish, try fish oil supplements. Keeping up your magnesium intake, with leafy green veg, Brazil nuts and a supplement if necessary, is also a good idea, as levels can be low in asthma sufferers and the mineral may be needed to help airways relax.

Limited evidence suggests pine bark extract (Pycnogenol) might be helpful, and the herb pelargonium is definitely one to watch, having been shown recently to ease symptoms of the chronic lung disease COPD (congestive obstructive pulmonary disease). For wheezing that only comes on after exercise, a large daily dose (1000mg) of vitamin C might help improve symptoms in some affected individuals.

CARDIOVASCULAR DISEASE

Death rates from heart disease and strokes have fallen considerably in recent years, but these cardiovascular diseases were still the biggest killers in statistics from 2010. Not smoking, keeping alcohol intake modest, and reducing salt and saturated fat intakes are key strategies to prevent both heart attack and stroke. Having a portion or two of oily fish weekly – or its equivalent in fish oils – provides heart-healthy omega-3s that can be protective too. For stroke protection, it appears that having lots of tomato lycopene might be useful too. Finnish researchers found that men with the greatest amounts of lycopene in their blood had a 55% lower chance of having any kind of stroke.

CIRCULATION (POOR)

Oily fish, garlic and plenty of fruit and veg will all stand you in good stead in terms of a healthy circulation, as they contain components that keep blood flowing and arteries healthy. Of the herbs and supplements available for boosting circulation, ginkgo is probably the best and most well known, and is worth trying if you suffer with general symptoms such as cold hands and feet. (See also 'Venous Insufficiency/Varicose Veins', page 118.)

COLDS AND MINOR INFECTIONS

Everyone gets colds and flu from time to time, but frequent infections may indicate that your immune system is struggling. Make sure your intake of vitamin A-rich foods such as carrot and peppers is adequate, as these maintain the mucous passages that keep out bacteria and viruses. Zinc, selenium and vitamin D play an important part in immunity, and it could be a good idea to take a multivitamin that contains all these to cover nutritional gaps or times when you are not eating as well as you should. If you're under lots of physical stress – if you do punishing workouts or work outside in extremes of temperature, for example – a 200mg vitamin C supplement may protect against the lowering effect that this stress has on the immune system. Try sucking zinc lozenges (according to the pack instructions) the minute you feel a cold coming on, or take a regular zinc-containing supplement every day as a preventative measure. Echinacea and pelargonium might also help.

CRAMPS

If your muscle cramps occur during sports activity, the most likely cause is not getting enough fluids, so do drink plenty whilst exercising and increase your potassium intake (orange juice and bananas are good sources). If it's hot or you're exercising for a prolonged time, consider sports drinks that replenish lost minerals too.

Calcium and magnesium are both important for correct muscle function, but there's little evidence that taking these will help with the nocturnal night cramps experienced by 60% of older people. However, a review by the Cochrane Library of magnesium and cramps concluded that magnesium might be potentially more useful in pregnancy-related muscle cramps and that more research is warranted in this area.

DEPRESSION

Poor diet can contribute to depression, but you can help improve your mental health by choosing fewer processed and high-sugar foods and drinks and more wholegrain cereals, pulses, fruit and vegetables, maintaining a healthy weight by exercising regularly, and watching your alcohol intake. Including protein at each meal so that your body can make a steady supply of serotonin is also important. Two supplements that may help – but only if your doctor has not already prescribed antidepressants – are 5-HTP and the traditional herbal medicine St John's wort, but only one or the other should be taken, not both.

DIABETES COMPLICATIONS

Diabetic neuropathy is a type of nerve damage associated with diabetes. It results in damage to the nerves in a person's feet, legs and eyes, and can have serious complications. Three natural supplements – alpha lipoic acid, acetyl-L-carnitine and evening primrose oil – have shown some promise for the damage to the nerves. For helping with diabetic retinopathy – another diabetes complication that results in damage to the back of the eye – pine bark extracts such as Pycnogenol may be useful. All complications of diabetes can be serious and should never be managed without the help of a diabetic specialist.

DVT

The scourge of modern life and long-haul flights, deep vein thrombosis (DVT) is when a dangerous clot forms in one of the deep veins of the body. Being overweight and very inactive are risk factors, as are smoking and a family history of thrombosis.

If you're going to travel on a long-haul flight or be laid up for a while, one thing you can try taking to reduce your risk of DVT is a patented extract from tomatoes called Fruitflow. This ingredient has been shown to dampen signals that cause blood platelets to stick together, preventing clots forming. The manufacturers have been allowed by the European Food Safety Authority to make a claim that Fruitflow 'helps maintain normal platelet aggregation, which contributes to healthy blood flow'. Studies suggest that it is effective an hour and a half after it's consumed and for up to 18 hours.

ERECTILE DYSFUNCTION

Erection difficulties should be explored medically, and any underlying psychological issues should be examined too. Losing weight, stopping smoking and cutting down on alcohol are key things to do. Supplement-wise, arginine, an amino acid found in protein foods, is a popular supplement, on the basis that it can stimulate nitric oxide, essential to the dilation of blood vessels that make an erection happen. Though it's likely that the bigger issue around erectile dysfunction and nitric oxide is not how much nitric oxide is produced by the body, but how sensitively the body reacts to it. Other research findings suggest that some men may find a supplement of Panax ginseng moderately helpful. However, it's important to know that there's no herb or supplement that is definitely proven to help erections and that products that claim to be aphrodisiac or to cure impotence are making false and misleading claims.

HAY FEVER

Diet and supplements can only ever play second fiddle to antihistamines, but there's certainly no harm in eating lots of quercetin-rich onions and/or taking a quercetin supplement, which has been shown in the laboratory to stop the production and release of histamine. Anecdotally, buying and eating local honey which contains traces of the pollens you come across every day helps some people (the theory being that you become desensitised to the traces of pollen allergens it contains). One small study suggests that the probiotic bacteria *Lactobacillus acidophilus* might help reduce allergic reaction to pollen, but this could be an anomaly unless confirmed by other studies. In terms of long-term hay-fever prevention, a study published in the journal *Thorax* found that Cretan children eating a Mediterranean diet rich in nuts, grapes, oranges, apples and fresh tomatoes were protected against wheezing and nasal congestion.

HIGH BLOOD PRESSURE

The main dietary measures needed to tackle high blood pressure involve reducing salt (sodium) intake from processed foods, and losing weight if necessary. Balancing lower sodium intakes with a higher intake of potassium and calcium will also help. The Dietary Approaches to Stop Hypertension (DASH) diet includes lots of whole grains, fruits, vegetables and low-fat dairy products and is a proven regime to reduce blood pressure. Foods like blueberries and other purple fruit that are very rich in anthocyanins may also help lower blood pressure.

HIGH CHOLESTEROL

Components of your diet that can actively lower cholesterol include soya protein (from edamame beans, tofu, soya milk, etc.) and plant sterols (used to fortify some yoghurts and spreads and also available in supplement form). The multi-factorial approach to lowering cholesterol that's embraced by the Heart UK-endorsed Ultimate Cholesterol Lowering Plan includes plant sterols, soya, nuts and a good source of soluble fibre, such as oats. Being a healthy weight and being physically active will also improve your cholesterol balance.

INFERTILITY

Infertility affects as many as one in six couples and in some cases improving diet may help. An eight-year study of more than 18,000 women uncovered several evidence-based suggestions for improved fertility that included getting more iron from plant sources (like cashews and watercress), avoiding trans fats (largely removed from supermarket food, but still found widely in fried takeaway foods in the UK), replacing a daily portion of meat protein with plant protein (such as tofu or quorn), and choosing slower energy-releasing carbohydrates such as whole grains, vegetables, whole fruits (not juices) and beans, that can improve blood sugar and insulin levels.

For men, particularly those with poor diets, a supplement of antioxidant vitamins and minerals may help (presumably by improving sperm quality). And both men and women can benefit by reducing alcohol intake and getting enough zinc, which is required for the health of both male and female reproductive organs. All women trying to get pregnant should take a daily 400 microgram folic acid supplement.

MENOPAUSAL SYMPTOMS

In South East Asia, women have fewer hot flushes than women in the West, and this has been linked with their higher consumption of the isoflavones (which have minor oestrogen-like effects) in soya foods. We don't know whether this is cause and effect, or if some other aspect of Asian women's lifestyles or genetic makeup brings about the benefit. Eating more soya foods can't do any harm though.

The traditional herbal medicine black cohosh could also help, and this is the time of life when women should start making sure they get high intakes of calcium and vitamin D for their bones too.

MIGRAINE

Many people find foods can trigger their migraine, but it's not necessarily always the stereotypical ones of chocolate, cheese, caffeine and red wine. To find out if there's a pattern, it's worth keeping a diet and symptom diary. However, aged and fermented foods, such as aged cheeses, smoked fish and cured meats, are generally agreed to be particular culprits.

As a long-term preventive for migraines, you might want to try the traditional herbal medicine feverfew; there's also some evidence that 5-HTP can help. Several studies also suggest that magnesium levels are lower in people with migraine, and a magnesium supplement could be useful for sufferers whose levels are low – particularly women who get menstrual migraines.

MOUTH ULCERS

Mouth ulcers can occur as a result of a physical trauma to the mouth (poorly fitting braces or dentures for example), but may be also stress and diet related. If you get frequent outbreaks, track what you eat, as chocolate, coffee, peanuts, almonds, strawberries, cheese, tomatoes and wheat flour can trigger outbreaks in some people. A deficiency of vitamin B12 is another trigger, but always see your doctor to discuss this possibility as significant vitamin B12 deficiency is often down to a problem with absorption of the vitamin, rather than not getting enough in your diet, so supplements might not help. Optimal levels of dietary zinc are useful in healing, and the best thing for regular mouth ulcers, as well as generally improving your diet, is to take a multivitamin.

OSTEOARTHRITIS

Losing any excess weight helps relieve the pressure on the joints, and may minimise the loss of cartilage and pain in this wear-and-tear type of arthritis. A diet that's Mediterranean in style (full of antioxidant-rich and anti-inflammatory foods like oily fish, colourful veg, pulses and nuts) gives just the nutritional support you need if you're battling painful joints. In addition, supplements that could be particularly worth trying in moderate or severe osteoarthritis are glucosamine and chondroitin combinations, bromelain and possibly turmeric. None is a miracle cure but if one or a combination can help you reduce your intake of pain-killing drugs it's a big bonus.

OSTEOPOROSIS

Osteoporosis is a bone-thinning disease which affects one in three women after the menopause and an increasing number of men. The disease is better prevented than treated, because once the symptoms appear, a lot of the bone mass has already been lost. Weight-bearing exercise, such as walking and jogging, can build bone mass early in life and prevent loss later on; hormone replacement therapy after the menopause is another option.

The main dietary measures that help are a high intake of calcium and vitamin D: it's recommended that women at high risk of osteoporosis get 800mg–1200mg of calcium a day, plus at least 10 micrograms of vitamin D. There is also evidence that having certain other minerals alongside these two, such as zinc, magnesium, manganese, boron, copper and selenium, can enhance the strength of bones. It's important to eat enough greens, as vitamin K also helps keep bones strong.

PREGNANCY PRE-ECLAMPSIA

There are no reliable guidelines to prevent pre-eclampsia, but eating regularly spaced healthy meals and taking a pregnancy vitamin supplement should help. Potential benefit has been shown in small studies that used lycopene and CoQ10, but if you're not at any known high risk of pre-eclampsia it wouldn't be recommended that you take these during pregnancy. Low calcium may be a different story however: calcium is a really important mineral during pregnancy, and studies show that women who have a low calcium intake but take calcium supplements may reduce their risk of pre-eclampsia, eclampsia and premature birth.

PREMENSTRUAL SYNDROME

This unpleasant collection of physical and emotional symptoms suffered by women in the days approaching a period may be helped by keeping blood sugar levels even with small, frequent meals, and by minimising intakes of sugar, salt and caffeine. Suggested supplements are up to 1000mg of calcium, which may decrease bloating, depression and aches, and up to 400mg of magnesium to help decrease pain and fluid retention, and to improve mood. Some women take evening primrose oil for breast tenderness, and some doctors also recommend up to 10mg of vitamin B6.

PROSTATE TROUBLES

Lots of men get prostate troubles as they get older, but all men who experience difficulty with urination should see a doctor. If the diagnosis is a benign enlargement of the prostate, the herb saw palmetto may be useful for dealing with mild urinary symptoms, as may a plant sterol called beta sitosterol, also available in supplement form. For prostatitis (inflammation of the prostate gland) there's preliminary evidence that a supplement of the flavonoid quercetin might help.

RHEUMATOID ARTHRITIS

Rheumatoid arthritis is an autoimmune condition in which the body's immune system attacks the joints. As with osteoarthritis, if you are overweight, losing weight can significantly reduce pain in the weight-bearing joints. Eating plenty of fruit and veg, plus oily fish or fish oil, which have anti-inflammatory properties, should help. It's also worth making sure you're getting enough selenium – an important antioxidant that may play a role in keeping joints healthy. Consuming too many omega-6 fats in margarines and vegetable oils may not be good for people with rheumatoid arthritis as it might increase inflammation, but GLA, an omega-6 fat found in evening primrose oil, is an exception.

TIREDNESS

General fatigue may be caused by several factors, the most likely of which are stress and lack of sleep. The commonest of the nutritional causes – though more likely in women than men – is iron deficiency. Many other marginal nutrient deficiencies could also potentially result in lowered energy levels, and a multivitamin and mineral supplement may help to lift fatigue that's linked to nutritional deficiency. Look for one with reasonably good levels of magnesium (say 25% of the RDA). Any ongoing tiredness that does not resolve itself through good nutrition, relaxation and a few good nights' sleep should be referred to a health professional.

VENOUS INSUFFICIENCY/VARICOSE VEINS

Venous insufficiency is the condition in which the tiny one-way valves in the leg veins that prevent blood falling back into the feet start to fail. Many people over 40 are affected and of these, 20–25% of the women and 10–15% of men will also have visible varicose veins. Pycnogenol has shown promise in reducing symptoms of venous insufficiency such as leg pain and swelling. In a review of studies by the Cochrane Library another traditional herbal medicine – horse chestnut extract – was also shown to help.

WOUND HEALING

Almost any aspect of a poorly balanced diet could affect wound healing, so a comprehensive A–Z multivitamin is a good idea. In particular, adequate levels of zinc (in lean red meat) and vitamin C (in citrus fruits) will help. As an added bonus, the flavonoids in citrus fruits have been shown to strengthen capillaries and reduce the risk of bruising. Some vitamin C supplements contain these flavonoids (also called bioflavonoids) in one handy package.

USEFUL RESOURCES

The following places are useful sources of further information.

NHS 'BEHIND THE NEWS'

From the NHS, this webpage digs behind the headlines of vitamin, nutrition and other general health stories you read in British newspapers.
www.nhs.uk/news

PATIENT.CO.UK

Lots of patient-focused information, including on some supplements.
www.patient.co.uk

HSIS

The website of the Health Supplements Information Service is funded by the Proprietary Association of Great Britain (PAGB) and companies that manufacture food supplements, but it still contains useful information on vitamins and minerals and how the industry in Europe is regulated.
www.hsis.org

OFFICE OF DIETARY SUPPLEMENTS

From the US National Institutes of Health, this official website of the Office of Dietary Supplements offers comprehensive overviews of vitamins, minerals and other supplements.
www.ods.od.nih.gov

OTHER WEBSITES

Some American universities or American university hospitals also produce very useful plain English reviews of the science behind supplements and healthy eating in general.

Harvard School of Public Health: www.hsph.harvard.edu/nutritionsource
University of Maryland: www.umm.edu/health
Tuft's Medial Center: www.tuftsmedicalcenter.org
University of California at Berkeley: www.berkeleywellness.com/supplements

INDEX